Chronic Hepatitis B: An Update

Guest Editor

NAOKY C.S. TSAI, MD

CLINICS IN LIVER DISEASE

www.liver.theclinics.com

Consulting Editor
NORMAN M. GITLIN, MD

August 2010 • Volume 14 • Number 3

SAUNDERS an imprint of ELSEVIER, Inc.

W.B. SAUNDERS COMPANY

A Division of Elsevier Inc.

1600 John F. Kennedy Boulevard, Suite 1800 ● Philadelphia, PA 19103-2899

http://www.theclinics.com

CLINICS IN LIVER DISEASE Volume 14, Number 3
August 2010 ISSN 1089-3261, ISBN-13: 978-1-4377-2532-2

Editor: Kerry Holland

Clinics in Liver Disease (ISSN 1089-3261) is published quarterly by Elsevier Inc., 360 Park Avenue South, New York, NY 10010-1710. Months of issue are February, May, August, and November. Business and Editorial Offices: 1600 John F. Kennedy Blvd., Ste. 1800, Philadelphia, PA 19103-2899. Customer Service Office: 3251 Riverport Lane, Maryland Heights, MO 63043. Periodicals postage paid at New York, NY and additional mailing offices. Subscription prices are $235.00 per year (U.S. individuals), $118.00 per year (U.S. student/resident), $340.00 per year (U.S. institutions), $311.00 per year (foreign individuals), $163.00 per year (foreign student/ resident), $409.00 per year (foreign instituitions), $271.00 per year (Canadian individuals), $163.00 per year (Canadian student/resident), and $409.00 per year (Canadian institutions). Foreign air speed delivery is included in all *Clinics* subscription prices. All prices are subject to change without notice. **POSTMASTER:** Send address changes to *Clinics in Liver Disease*, Elsevier Health Sciences Division, Subscription Customer Service, 3251 Riverport Lane, Maryland Heights, MO 63043. **Customer Service: Telephone: 1-800-654-2452 (U.S. and Canada); 314-447-8871 (outside U.S. and Canada). Fax: 314-447-8029. E-mail: journalscustomer service-usa@elsevier.com (for print support); journalsonlinesupport-usa@elsevier.com (for online support).**

Reprints. For copies of 100 or more of articles in this publication, please contact the Commercial Reprints Department, Elsevier Inc., 360 Park Avenue South, New York, NY 10010-1710. Tel.: 212-633-3812; Fax: 212-462-1935; E-mail: reprints@elsevier.com.

Clinics in Liver Disease is covered in *MEDLINE/PubMed (Index Medicus)*.

Printed and bound by CPI Group (UK) Ltd, Croydon, CR0 4YY

Transferred to Digital Print 2011

Contributors

CONSULTING EDITOR

NORMAN M. GITLIN, MD, FRCP(London), FRCPE(Edinburgh), FACG, FACP
Formerly, Professor of Medicine, Chief of Hepatology, Emory University; Currently, Consultant, Atlanta Gastroenterology Associates, Atlanta, Georgia

GUEST EDITOR

NAOKY C.S. TSAI, MD
Professor of Medicine, John A. Burns School of Medicine, Hawaii, Manoa Liver Center, Hawaii Medical Center, Honolulu, Hawaii

AUTHORS

SCOTT BOWDEN, PhD
Associate Professor, Department of Molecular Microbiology, Victorian Infectious Diseases Reference Laboratory, North Melbourne, Victoria, Australia

CORINNE BUCHANAN, MSN, ACNP-BC
Center for Liver Transplantation, Cedars-Sinai Medical Center, Los Angeles, California

KYONG-MI CHANG, MD
Associate Professor of Medicine, Division of Gastroenterology, Philadelphia Veterans Affairs Medical Center; University of Pennsylvania School of Medicine, Philadelphia, Pennsylvania

MEI HWEI CHANG, MD
Professor, Department of Pediatrics; Chairman, Hepatitis Research Center, National Taiwan University Hospital, College of Medicine, National Taiwan University, Taipei, Taiwan

EDWARD C. DOO, MD
Program Director, Liver Diseases Research Branch, Division of Digestive Diseases and Nutrition, National Institute of Diabetes and Digestive and Kidney Diseases, National Institutes of Health, Bethesda, Maryland

MARC G. GHANY, MD, MHSc
Staff Physician, Liver Diseases Branch, National Institute of Diabetes and Digestive and Kidney Diseases, National Institutes of Health, Bethesda, Maryland

STEVEN-HUY B. HAN, MD, AGAF
Professor of Medicine and Surgery, Dumont-UCLA Liver Transplant Center, David Geffen School of Medicine at University of California, Los Angeles, Los Angeles, California

SYED-MOHAMMED R. JAFRI, MD
Hepatology Fellow, Division of Gastroenterology, University of Michigan Health System, Ann Arbor, Michigan

MICHELLE LAI, MD, MPH
Instructor in Medicine, Department of Medicine, Division of Gastroenterology, Beth Israel Deaconess Medical Center, Harvard University, Boston, Massachusetts

YUN-FAN LIAW, MD
Professor of Medicine, Liver Research Unit, Chang Gung Memorial Hospital, Chang Gung University College of Medicine, Taipei, Taiwan

STEPHEN LOCARNINI, MBBS, PhD, FRC[Path]
Professor, Head of R&MD, Victorian Infectious Diseases Reference Laboratory, North Melbourne, Victoria, Australia

ANNA SUK-FONG LOK, MD
Alice Lohrman Andrews Research Professor in Hepatology; Director of Clinical Hepatology; Associate Chair for Clinical Research, Department of Internal Medicine, Division of Gastroenterology, University of Michigan Health System, Ann Arbor, Michigan

PAUL MARTIN, MD, FRCP, FRCPI
Professor of Medicine and Chief, Division of Hepatology, Schiff Liver Institute, Center for Liver Diseases, University of Miami Miller School of Medicine, Miami, Florida

AMY C. MCCLUNE, MD
Assistant Professor of Medicine and Surgery, David Geffen School of Medicine at University of California, Los Angeles, The Pfleger Liver Institute, Los Angeles, California

BRIAN J. MCMAHON, MD
Liver Disease and Hepatitis Program, Alaska Native Tribal Health Consortium; Arctic Investigations Program, Centers for Disease Control and Prevention, Anchorage, Alaska

HUI-HUI TAN, MBBS, MRCP
Consultant, Department of Gastroenterology and Hepatology, Singapore General Hospital, Singapore, Singapore

MYRON J. TONG, MD, PhD
Professor of Medicine and Surgery, David Geffen School of Medicine at University of California, Los Angeles, The Pfleger Liver Institute, Los Angeles, California

TRAM T. TRAN, MD
Medical Director, Center for Liver Transplantation, Cedars-Sinai Medical Center; Associate Professor of Medicine, Geffen University of California, Los Angeles, School of Medicine, Los Angeles, California

HANK S. WANG, MD
Fellow, Division of Digestive Diseases, Dumont-UCLA Liver Transplant Center, David Geffen School of Medicine at University of California Los Angeles, Los Angeles, California

Contents

> In this article, the 4 phases of chronic HBV infection are reviewed and the factors that are associated with disease progression and the development of hepatocellular carcinoma (HCC) and cirrhosis are discussed. Also discussed is what is known to date about how to identify persons at the highest risk of developing HCC and/or cirrhosis. Finally, ways in which the natural history can be altered by hepatitis B vaccination and identification, close monitoring, and appropriate treatment of chronically infected individuals are reviewed.

> A basic understanding of the molecular events involved in the hepatitis B virus (HBV) life cycle is essential to better appreciate the natural history and atypical presentations of the disease and to develop individual management plans based on readily available virologic tests. With the improved knowledge gained from studying the molecular biology of HBV, novel approaches to inhibition of viral replication are being explored, such as viral entry inhibitors, nucleocapsid inhibitors, and inhibitors of viral assembly. However, the ultimate goal of therapy is to identify strategies to eliminate covalently closed circular DNA from infected hepatocytes. This article serves to introduce the clinically relevant aspects of the HBV life cycle as they pertain to patient management.

> Hepatitis B virus (HBV) is a hepatotrophic DNA virus that causes acute and chronic hepatitis. Despite an effective vaccine, more than 350 million people are chronically infected with HBV worldwide and are at risk for progressive liver disease. There are marked geographic variations in HBV prevalence (ranging from 0.1% to 2% in low prevalence areas and 10% to 20% in high prevalence areas) related to the timing and mode of HBV exposure. In many developed countries, HBV exposure typically occurs in adults via sexual transmission with a low chronicity rate (5%). In regions with high HBV prevalence (eg, Asia, sub-Saharan Africa), HBV exposure tends to occur in the perinatal period (eg, vertical transmission from mother to infant) with a high rate of persistence in the absence of timely vaccination. The course of viral infection is defined by the interplay between the virus and host immune defense. This article

introduces the innate and adaptive immune defense mechanisms in general and as related to HBV. In particular, the current concepts regarding the innate and adaptive immune components contributing to the clinical, virologic and therapeutic outcome in acute and chronic hepatitis B are examined.

The goal of antiviral therapy for chronic hepatitis B is to prevent the development of cirrhosis and hepatocellular carcinoma. End points, including viral suppression, alanine aminotransferase normalization, hepatitis B e antigen loss, hepatitis B surface antigen loss, and improvement in liver histology, are used to determine treatment success. Treatment is based on hepatitis B virus (HBV) replication status and stage of liver disease, modulated by the age of the patient, hepatitis B e antigen (HBeAg) status and patient preference. Seven therapies are approved, including two formulations of interferon and five orally administered nucleos(t)ide analogs. These therapies are effective in suppressing HBV replication and have also been shown to prevent disease progression.

The introduction of nucleos(t)ide analog therapy has seen the emergence of antiviral drug resistance, which has become the main factor limiting the long-term application of these antiviral agents for patients with chronic hepatitis B. The prevention of resistance requires the adoption of strategies that effectively control virus replication and exploit an understanding of the mechanisms and processes that drive the emergence of drug resistance, namely high replication rates, low fidelity of the hepatitis B virus rt/polymerase, selective pressure of the nucleos(t)ide analog, role of replication space (liver turnover), fitness of the mutant, and genetic barrier to the drug.

Hepatocellular carcinoma (HCC) is the fifth most common cancer in the world and the third leading cause of cancer-related deaths. More than 80% of HCC cases are from the Asian and African continents, and more than 50% of cases are from mainland China. Approximately 350 million to 400 million persons are chronically infected with hepatitis B virus (HBV), and this virus is the most common cause of HCC worldwide. It is estimated that more than 50% of liver cancers worldwide are attributable to HBV and up to 89% of HBV-related HCC are from developing countries. Recently, increasing trends in HCC incidence have been reported from several Western countries, including France, Australia, and the United States.

The consequences of chronic hepatitis B virus infection include hepatocellular carcinoma and liver cirrhosis. Effective antiviral therapy in patients with hepatitis B with advanced liver disease with viral suppression and sustained HBeAg seroconversion (where applicable) may abort hepatic decompensation, diminish hepatocellular risk, and reduce the risk of viral recurrence after transplantation. Overt hepatic decompensation is an indication for referral to a transplant center.

Providing appropriate treatment and follow-up to hepatitis B virus (HBV)–infected mothers and their newborns is critical in preventing HBV mother-to-child transmission (MTCT) and eradicating HBV infection. Although highly effective in preventing MTCT, standard passive-active immunoprophylaxis with hepatitis B immunoglobulin and the hepatitis B vaccine may have a failure rate as high as 10% to 15%. Antiviral treatment has been used during pregnancy and may decrease MTCT. Several issues must be addressed in future clinical studies before universal recommendations for antiviral therapy for pregnant women can be made.

Hepatitis B virus is a common cause of acute liver failure. It can be especially problematic in patients coinfected with hepatitis C, hepatitis D or human immunodeficiency virus. In addition, immunosuppression-associated hepatitis B reactivation is being increasingly recognized following chemotherapy, biologic therapy, and organ transplantation. This article highlights treatment options in these special populations.

Prevention is most cost effective toward successful control of hepatitis B virus (HBV) infection and its complications. It is particularly urgent where HBV infection and hepatocellular carcinoma (HCC) are prevalent. To achieve better results of primary HCC prevention globally, higher world coverage rates of HBV vaccine, better strategies against breakthrough infection/nonresponder, and good long-term protection are needed. With the universal hepatitis B vaccination program starting from neonates in most countries, HBV infection and its complications will be further reduced in this century. An effective decline in the incidence of HCC in adults is expected in the near future. The concept of a cancer preventive vaccine, using HBV as an example, can be applied further to other infectious agents and their related cancers.

There have been major advances in the field of hepatitis B (HBV) over the last few decades. These advances have resulted in the understanding of the natural history of chronic HBV infection, effective vaccines against the virus, sensitive assays for screening and monitoring of treatment, and effective treatments for viral suppression, all leading to improved outcomes. Debates and controversies remain, however, over the ideal management strategies of patients with chronic hepatitis B. To eradicate HBV, the global community needs to improve current preventive, screening, and treatment strategies.

THE CLINICS ARE NOW AVAILABLE ONLINE!

Access your subscription at:
www.theclinics.com

Preface

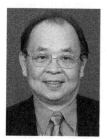

Naoky C.S. Tsai, MD
Guest Editor

It has been more than 4 decades since Australian antigen was discovered by Drs Blumberg, Alter, and their colleagues in 1967. During the subsequent decades of remarkable discoveries, hepatitis B virus was identified and its molecular structures, genome and life cycle, natural history of the chronic infection, and connection with chronic hepatitis and hepatocellular carcinoma were well characterized and understood. Based on this knowledge, an effective and safe vaccine was developed, which was later declared as the first cancer-preventing vaccine by the World Health Organization. With the understanding of its life cycle, a class of safe and effective, although not perfect, antiviral therapies had become available, which showed promising results in suppressing the hepatitis viral replication and, in turn, altering the natural history of this disease in patients with advanced liver disease.

Now in 2010, we should be reaping the benefit of these discoveries. Yet several studies have shown that there is still a wide gap in access to care for those with chronic infection. Less than 10% of the 1.25 million people estimated by the Centers for Disease Control and Prevention to be chronically infected are under medical management. Even more people are unexposed yet unvaccinated, despite a national universal vaccination program started in early 1990s in the United States. Although many reasons are behind these discrepancies, a recent Institute of Medicine report concludes, "there is a lack of knowledge and awareness about chronic viral hepatitis on the part of health care and social-service providers, as well as among at-risk populations, members of the public, and policy-makers. Due to the insufficient understanding about the extent and seriousness of this public-health problem, inadequate public resources are being allocated to prevention, control, and surveillance programs." With these concerns in mind, the primary goal of this issue of *Clinics in Liver Disease* is to assemble a group of experts in this field to present their expertise knowledge at such a level where practicing clinicians who deal with this disease in their daily practice can understand it and thereby implement this knowledge into their own practice. Briefly, in this issue of the *Clinics in Liver Disease*, Dr Brian McMahon discusses the natural history of chronic hepatitis B using his vast knowledge and

Clin Liver Dis 14 (2010) xi–xii
doi:10.1016/j.cld.2010.05.011
1089-3261/10/$ – see front matter © 2010 Elsevier Inc. All rights reserved.

liver.theclinics.com

experience from working with a highly endemic population of Inuit in Alaska; Drs Marc Ghany and Edward Doo give an easy-to-understand description of hepatitis B virus (HBV) virology; Dr Kyon-Mi Chang discusses HBV immunology, which is the least understood area of this disease but has the most potential to improve knowledge in the management of chronic hepatitis B; Dr Anna Lok gives her authoritative review on the current issues and controversies of treatment of chronic hepatitis B; Dr Stephen Locarnini has extensive experience in antiviral resistance and its management, an important issue in the use of currently available antiviral oral agents; Dr Myron Tong discusses the current understanding of HBV carcinogenesis and updates on surveillance and treatment of hepatocellular carcinoma—the most dreadful outcome of this disease; Dr Paul Martin discusses management of end-stage chronic hepatitis B—antiviral therapy, monotherapy versus combotherapy, choice of agent, when to start therapy, and post-transplant patients, including duration of hepatitis B immune globulin therapy, HBcAb(+)-only recipients, and occult HBV infection; Dr Tram Tran discusses the treatment in reproductive women and during pregnancy and prevention of vertical transmission in third trimester with antiviral agents—an area with significant lack of good clinical evidence; Dr Steve Han discusses management of patients with acute hepatitis B, co-infection with hepatitis D virus/hepatitis C virus/HIV, and preimmunosuppressive therapy and management of renal and heart transplant patients with HBV infection; Dr Mei Huei Chang discusses Taiwanese success in implementing universal vaccination, leading to a remarkable reduction in prevalence of chronic hepatitis B and incidence of hepatocellular carcinoma; and, finally, Drs Michelle Lai and Yun Fan Liaw give a rundown of what has been accomplished and the hope for the future in the fight to control this disease. I would like to also acknowledge that almost all articles were coauthored by a young investigator.

Hepatitis B infection is a complicated illness, and I believe we will gain more knowledge into this disease, particularly with the recently launched Hepatitis B Research Network sponsored by National Institutes of Health–National Institute of Diabetes and Digestive and Kidney Diseases. Furthermore, newer highly effective vaccination can be developed, and novel treatments are being investigated. I have high hopes that with appropriate resources invested, this preventable disease can be eradicated from the world as were smallpox and polio.

Naoky C.S. Tsai, MD
Department of Medicine, John A. Burns School of Medicine, University of Hawaii
Manoa Liver Center, Hawaii Medical Center
East 2230 Liliha Street, MA 2nd Floor
Honolulu, HI 96734, USA

E-mail address:
naoky@hawaii.edu

Natural History of Chronic Hepatitis B

Brian J. McMahon, MD[a,b,*]

KEYWORDS

- Hepatitis B virus • Natural history • Hepatitis B genotypes
- Hepatocellular carcinoma

Hepatitis B virus (HBV) is the cause of one of the most common chronic viral infections in the world. More than 2 billion persons have been exposed to HBV and 350 to 400 million persons have chronic HBV infection.[1] The natural history of chronic HBV does not always progress in a linear fashion. Patients can go from a state of high viral levels and no liver disease activity to one of active liver disease, then to one of no liver activity with low viral levels.[2] However, reversions and reactivations can happen without warning, making management of HBV a real challenge. In this article, I review the 4 phases of chronic HBV infection and discuss the factors that are associated with disease progression and the development of hepatocellular carcinoma (HCC) and cirrhosis. Factors identified with these adverse outcomes (HCC and cirrhosis) are discussed including the role of HBV and (1) demographic features such as age and sex; (2) viral characteristics including HBV genotype, co-infections with other viruses, specific HBV viral mutations, and HBV DNA levels over time; and (3) social and environmental factors including alcohol, coffee, tobacco, and environmental toxins. I also touch on what is known to date about how to identify persons at the highest risk of developing HCC and/or cirrhosis. Finally, I discuss ways in which the natural history can be altered by hepatitis B vaccination and identification, close monitoring, and appropriate treatment of chronically infected individuals.

RISK OF DEVELOPING CHRONIC HBV AFTER ACUTE INFECTION

Several prospective population-based cohort studies have been conducted that have clearly identified younger age at infection as the strongest factor associated with the development of chronic HBV infection after acute exposure to the virus. The classic study by Palmer Beasley and collegues[3] in Taiwan showed that infants whose mothers

Funding Support: None.

[a] Liver Disease and Hepatitis Program, Alaska Native Tribal Health Consortium, Anchorage, AK, USA

[b] Arctic Investigations Program, Centers for Disease Control and Prevention, Anchorage, AK, USA

* 4315 Diplomacy Drive, Anchorage, AK 99508.

E-mail address: bdm9@cdc.gov

Clin Liver Dis 14 (2010) 381–396

doi:10.1016/j.cld.2010.05.007

1089-3261/10/$ – see front matter © 2010 Elsevier Inc. All rights reserved.

liver.theclinics.com

were positive for hepatitis B surface antigen (HBsAg), the marker for active HBV infection, and also positive for hepatitis B "e" antigen (HBeAg), a marker for high viral load, had virtually 100% risk of being infected with HBV at or near the time of birth; whereas icteric hepatitis was rare, 90% of these infants developed chronic HBV infection. Fortunately, administration of hepatitis B immune globulin (HBIG) and hepatitis B vaccine at birth could reduce this risk of chronicity to less than 5%.[4] Those infants whose mothers were negative for HBeAg and positive for HBsAg plus antibody to hepatitis B "e" antigen (anti-HBe) had an only 15% chance of developing chronic HBV infection if they did not receive hepatitis B vaccine with or without HBIG, but had a slight chance of having acute icteric hepatitis B. One study from Africa showed that children born without HBV but infected during the first 2 years of life had a 50% chance of becoming chronically infected.[5] Two prospective studies, one in Taiwan and one in Alaska, of children infected after birth but before 5 years of age showed that approximately 30% developed chronic HBV.[6,7] However, prospective studies performed in persons infected when older than 10 years of age showed that fewer than 10% became chronically infected whereas up to 30% had acute icteric infection.[7] **Table 1** summarizes the risk of developing chronic HBV after acquisition by age.

RISK OF HEPATOCELLULAR CARCINOMA AND CIRRHOSIS

Prospective population-based cohort studies have clearly shown an increased risk of HCC in patients with chronic HBV infection.[8,9] Because most persons with chronic HBV infection are asymptomatic, population estimates of the risk of developing cirrhosis would be dependent on population-based liver biopsy studies that included liver biopsies of all infected persons regardless of clinical status, which for obvious ethical reasons have not been done. However, the incidence of decompensated cirrhosis in chronic HBsAg-positive carriers has been shown to be approximately 0.5 per 1000 person years in population-based studies, to as high as 2% to 3% per year in clinic-based longitudinal studies, the higher percentage in clinic-based studies likely attributable to referral bias.[9–14] In persons with HBV who are found to have compensated cirrhosis on liver biopsy, the survival rate was 84% and 68% at 5 and

Table 1
The risk of developing chronic hepatitis B infection after acute exposure

Mode of Transmission	Age at Infection	Risk of Acute Icteric Hepatitis	Risk of Chronic HBV Infection	Lifetime Risk of HCC[a]
Perinatal HBeAg-positive mother	Birth	<1%	90%	15%–40%
Perinatal HBeAg-negative mother	Birth	5%	<15%	15%–40%
Horizontal	Between birth and age 2 years	<10%	50%	15%–40%
Horizontal	2–5 years	9%	30%	15%–25%
Horizontal	5–10 years	10%	16%	15%–25%
Horizontal	>10 years	10%–33%	7%–14%	Unknown

[a] In those with chronic HBV infection.

10 years respectively, but for those who presented with decompensated cirrhosis before the availability of oral antiviral agents, the 5-year survival rate was found to be only 14%.[15–17]

PHASES OF CHRONIC HEPATITIS B INFECTION

The National Institutes of Health, at a workshop in 2007 and a consensus conference in 2008, identified 4 phases of HBV infection: the immune-tolerant phase, the immune-active phase, the inactive phase, and the so called "resolution phase" (**Table 2**).[18,19] The evolution of persons through the phases of chronic HBV infection is displayed in **Fig. 1**. The immune-tolerant phase predominantly occurs in persons infected at birth through perinatal transmission of HBV from mothers who are HBeAg antigen positive and is uncommon in children infected after birth. It predominately occurs in persons infected with HBV genotype C but can occur in those infected with other HBV genotypes. The median age when persons seroconvert from HBeAg to anti-HBe is in the fourth decade of life for those infected with HBV genotype C, whereas it occurs before age 20 years in those infected with other HBV genotypes.[20] Thus, most women infected with genotype C will remain HBeAg-positive throughout most of their child-bearing years, whereas those infected with other HBV genotypes will likely seroconvert much earlier in life. During the immune-tolerant phase, persons have very high levels of HBV DNA, usually more than 10 million IU/mL, and have normal alanine aminotransferase (ALT) levels with no or minimal liver inflammation or fibrosis on liver biopsy. In this phase, the immune system does not recognize HBV and there is no cytotoxic T-cell activity against the virus.[21] This phase may last more than 40 years in many persons infected at birth, especially if they have HBV genotype C infection.[20]

Most persons in the immune-tolerant phase will eventually go into the HBeAg-positive immune active phase as they age and recognize the virus as foreign. During this phase, ALT levels are elevated; HBV DNA levels are also elevated but lower than in the immune-tolerant phase, and active liver disease is found on biopsy. As this phase evolves, most often HBV DNA levels progressively fall, a weak cytotoxic T-cell response becomes active that eventually may get strong enough to suppress HBV DNA levels, and HBeAg seroconversion can occur. Once HBV seroconversion occurs, there can be 3 possible scenarios. From 10% to 40% of persons, varying by HBV genotype, can experience one or more reversions back to HBeAg seropositivity often associated with a flare of hepatitis that is usually subclinical and may not be noticed by the patient.[9,20] HBeAg seroreversions are seen more frequently in persons infected with HBV genotypes C or F.[20] These seroreversions tend to decrease in frequency over time and eventually stop.[9] A second possible outcome is that persons may

Table 2
Phases of chronic hepatitis B infection

HBV Phase	HBeAg	HBV DNA Level	Liver Biopsy Inflammation and Fibrosis
Immune tolerant	Positive	>200,000 IU/mL	None to minimal
Immune active	Positive or negative[a]	>20,000 IU/mL	Mild to severe
Inactive	Negative	<2,000 IU/mL	None to mild[b]
HBsAg clearance	Negative	<2,000 IU/mL	None to mild[b]

[a] Immune active phase may occasionally occur in persons with HBV DNA between 2000 and 20,000 IU/mL.
[b] May have moderate or severe fibrosis that may take years to resolve.

Natural Progression of HBV Infection

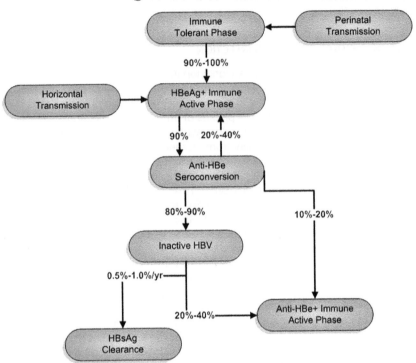

Fig. 1. A schematic algorithm to display the evolution of progression through the phases of hepatitis B virus infection. (*From* Goldstein ST, Zhou FJ, Hadler SC, et al. A mathematical model to estimate global hepatitis B disease burden and vaccination impact. Int J Epidemiol 2005;34(6):1329–39; with permission.)

remain in the immune-active phase even though they are HBeAg-negative/anti-HBe-positive. This is thought to occur in about 20% of persons after HBeAg seroconversion. These persons usually have an HBV DNA level higher than 20,000 IU/mL as well as an elevated ALT level, but occasionally persons with HBV DNA levels between 2000 and 20,000 IU/mL may have active hepatitis and fibrosis on liver biopsy.

Most persons after seroconversion experience a third outcome: what is termed the "inactive hepatitis B phase." This phase is characterized by HBeAg negativity, normal ALT, and HBV DNA levels that are below 2000 IU/mL and often undetectable by polymerase chain reaction (PCR) assay. Most patients remain in this inactive phase and may do so for life.[22,23] One study from Italy of 40 HBV-infected persons who remained in the inactive phase found that none of those without cirrhosis developed HCC, liver decompensation, or liver-related death over a median of 25 years and, of those with cirrhosis, none developed liver decompensation but 2 developed HCC.[12] During this phase, liver inflammation improves and may disappear and fibrosis reverses over time. Persons who remain in this phase usually have a more vigorous cytotoxic T-cell response directed at HBV.[21] Persons who undergo liver biopsy within a couple of years after going into the inactive HBV phase may still have minimal inflammation and substantial fibrosis that may take several years to reverse if the individual remains in the inactive carrier phase. These persons may be mistaken for individuals with active disease who need antiviral therapy, when in reality, their liver fibrosis is improving on its own. Clinicians should suspect this possibility when ALT is persistently normal and HBV DNA levels are low, and thereafter should follow these patients closely to make sure they stay in the inactive phase and not immediately put them on antiviral therapy unless they have bridging fibrosis or cirrhosis. It is important to remember that not all persons in the inactive phase remain there for life. An estimated 20% of them will reactivate to the HBeAg-negative or HBeAg-positive immune active phase and can experience recurring periods of reactivation and inactivation throughout their lives, which can lead to cirrhosis or HCC. This is why persons in the inactive HBV phase must be followed every 6 to 12 months for life with ALT levels because there are no predictors currently known as to who will remain in the inactive phase or revert to HBeAg-negative active hepatitis.

Some persons in the inactive phase will eventually clear HBsAg; most, but not all, will develop anti-HBs. In several large cohorts of HBV chronically infected persons the annual clearance of HBsAg ranged between 0.5% and 0.8% per year.[24–26] Factors associated with HBsAg clearance include older age but not sex or HBV genotype. Some refer to this as the "resolution phase" of HBV. Although the risk of cirrhosis appears to be very low after spontaneous HBsAg clearance, the risk of HCC is reduced but still significant, and has been reported in at least 6 studies.[24,25,27–29] In a study in Alaska of 1271 persons with chronic HBV infection followed prospectively for 20 years, the incidence of HCC after clearance of HBsAg was 36.8 compared with 195.7 per 100,000 person years of follow-up ($P<.001$).[26] Although this is a substantial reduction in risk, there still is a much higher risk of HCC than in the general population. In addition, the study from Alaska showed that most persons who developed HCC after HBsAg clearance and continued to undergo surveillance had their tumors detected at a resectable stage and 2 were long-term tumor-free survivors.[26] Thus, clinicians should consider having persons who were chronically infected and cleared HBsAg undergo surveillance for HCC, especially if they have risk factors such as presence of cirrhosis before HBsAg clearance, family history of HCC, or are males older than 40 years or females older than 50 years, even though surveillance is only recommended for HBsAg-positive persons by the American Association for the Study of Liver Diseases (AASLD) Practice Guideline for HCC.[30] Because the risk of HCC is still substantial, the name of this phase of chronic HBV infection should be changed from the "resolution phase" to the "HBsAg clearance phase." It is very possible that most persons with so-called "occult HBV" who are anti-HBc-positive but HBsAg-negative and develop HCC are really persons who previously had chronic HBV infection and cleared HBsAg.[26]

RISK FACTORS FOR DEVELOPING HCC AND CIRRHOSIS

The risk factors that have been identified that are associated with development of HCC are listed in **Tables 3** and **4**. These can be divided into demographic, viral, environmental, and socioeconomic. Under demographic, males have an increased risk of HCC over females of 3 or 4 to 1. The risk of HCC and cirrhosis is low before the age of 40 then rises exponentially with increasing age after the fourth decade of life (**Fig. 2**).[8,9,31] Also, there is an especially higher risk of HCC in persons with a family history of HCC.[32,33]

Environmental and social factors that increase the risk of HCC include heavy alcohol usage, smoking, and exposure to aflatoxin. Case-control studies have shown that heavy alcohol use increases the risk of both HCC and cirrhosis. Aflatoxins, a group of mycotoxins produced by the fungi *Aspergillus flavus* and *Aspergillus parasiticus* are molds found on grains and other foods in many nations, especially Africa and

Table 3
Demographic, social, and environmental risk factors associated with the development of hepatocellular carcinoma (HCC) and/or cirrhosis in persons with chronic hepatitis B virus infection

Demographic	Increased Risk of HCC	Increased Risk of Cirrhosis
Male sex	3+	+
Increasing age >40 years	3+	3+
Family history of HCC	3+	+
Social and environmental		
Alcohol	+	+
Aflatoxin	3+	Unknown
Smoking	+	+
Steatosis, metabolic syndrome, diabetes	No association	No association
Coffee	Decreased risk of HCC	Slower progression of liver fibrosis

Asia.[34] Aflatoxins are proven carcinogens that exert their influence on hepatocytes by inducing mutations in a variety of ways including at P53.[35] Exposure to aflatoxin is synergistic with HBV and greatly increases the risk of developing this cancer.[34,35] Smoking has been found to be a risk factor for HCC. Although the presence of the metabolic syndrome, obesity, elevated lipids and diabetes, and the presence of steatosis on liver biopsy are strongly associated with increased risk of liver fibrosis in HCV infection, the data are scanty in chronic HBV infection.[36] To date, most studies show no association between diabetes, the metabolic syndrome, or steatosis in persons with chronic HBV infection nor show increased risk of liver fibrosis on biopsy or subsequent development of HCC.[37–40] Multiple case-control and population-based studies have shown that coffee intake is inversely associated with cirrhosis and HCC. More specifically, it was recently shown in a prospective cohort study, the Hepatitis C Long-Term Treatment Against Cirrhosis (HALT-C) trial, that increasing coffee intake was associated with a lower rate of fibrosis progression defined by a 2-point change in the Ishak Fibrosis score.[41] Thus, increasing coffee intake appears to be a protective factor for progressive liver fibrosis in hepatitis C. This finding will need to be confirmed in HBV; however, because multiple studies have shown coffee intake to be protective in a variety of liver diseases, it may well also be protective in HBV.

Several viral factors have been associated with risk of liver disease progression and HCC. They include HBeAg positivity or high HBV viral load in persons older than 40 years, HBV genotypes C and F, basal core promoter (BCP) double mutation, and co-infection with other viruses. Several studies have demonstrated that persons older than 40 years with a high viral load and an HBV DNA higher than 20,000 IU/mL that remains elevated over time have a significantly increased risk of developing HCC when compared with persons with HBV DNA lower than 2000 IU/mL.[42–45] The most compelling of these is the Risk Evaluation of Viral Load Elevation and Associated Liver Disease/Cancer-Hepatitis B Virus (REVEAL-HBV) study, a population-based study of 3653 HBsAg-positive persons found from screening 28,870 individuals in 10 townships in Taiwan. The mean age of the cohort was 46 years at study entry and follow-up was for a mean of 11 years. HBV DNA was tested on entry and again at the end of the study only in those with an HBV DNA higher than 10^4 copies/mL (approximately 2000 IU/mL) at study entry. Those persons with HBV DNA levels higher

Table 4
Hepatitis B virus genotypes/subgenotypes: geographic regions and liver-related disease association

Genotype	Geographic Region	HBV Disease Association
A1	Central and eastern sub-Sahara Africa	HCC in young males
A2	Northern Europe	HCC and cirrhosis in older persons
A3	West Africa	HCC
B1	Japan	HCC and cirrhosis in older persons
B2-5, B7	East Asia	HCC and cirrhosis occur at younger age than B1
B6	Indigenous Populations in Alaska, Canada, Greenland	No serious sequelae identified to date
C1	Vietnam, Thailand, Myanmar, Indonesia	High rates of HCC and cirrhosis
C2	China, Taiwan, Korea, Japan	High rates of HCC and cirrhosis
C3	Pacific Islands (Micronesia, Melanesia, and Polynesia)	High rates of HCC and cirrhosis
D1	Europe, Middle East, Egypt, India, Asia	HBeAg-negative chronic hepatitis/cirrhosis and HCC
D2	Europe, Japan	HBeAg-negative chronic hepatitis/cirrhosis and HCC
D3	Europe, Asia, South Africa, United States	HBeAg-negative chronic hepatitis/cirrhosis and HCC
D4	Australia, Japan, Papua New Guinea	Not studied
E	West Africa	Not studied but area of high incidence of HCC
F1	Alaska, Argentina, Bolivia	HCC in young patients in Alaska
F2	Venezuela, Brazil	Fulminant hepatitis with HDV co-infection
F3	Venezuela, Columbia, Panama	Fulminant hepatitis with HDV co-infection
F4	Argentina	Not studied
G	France, United States, Vietnam	Usually found in co-infection with genotype A; increased association with acute hepatitis, liver fibrosis, and HCC in Vietnam
H	Mexico, Nicaragua, California	Not studied

Abbreviations: HCC, hepatocellular carcinoma; HBeAg, hepatitis B "e" antigen; HDV, hepatitis D virus.
Data from McMahon BJ. The influence of hepatitis B virus genotype and subgenotype on the natural history of chronic hepatitis B. Hepatol Int 2009;3(2):334–42.

than 10^4 copies/mL at entry that increased to higher than 10^5 copies/mL (approximately 20,000 IU/mL) at the end of the 11 years of follow-up were found to have a significantly higher risk of developing HCC during the study period than those with an initial level of HBV DNA of lower than 10^4 copies/mL at entry. Likewise, the incidence of cirrhosis was found to be significantly associated with HBV DNA levels higher than 10^4 copies/mL at study entry. Both of these findings were independent of ALT

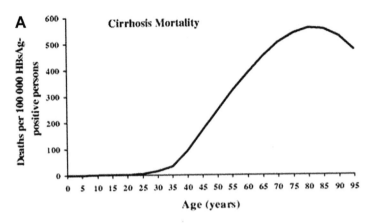

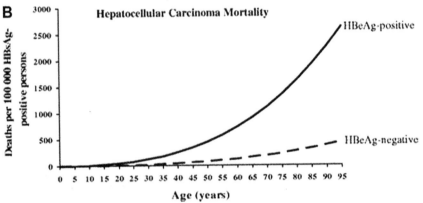

Fig. 2. A mathematical model displaying the global estimates of age-specific hepatitis B–related cirrhosis and hepatocellular carcinoma mortality. (*Adapted from* McMahon BJ. The natural history of chronic hepatitis B virus infection. Hepatology 2009;49:S45–S555; with permission.)

levels. This important study and the other population-based studies cited highlight the clinically important point that persons with HBV DNA higher than 20,000 IU/mL who are older than 40 years, especially those who are still HBeAg-positive, need very careful evaluation for the development of fibrosis as well as surveillance for HCC and intervention with antiviral therapy when appropriate, as recommended by established practice guidelines.[46] To date, there is no evidence that those persons who are younger than 40 years and have elevated levels of HBV DNA or are HBeAg-positive and have normal ALT levels, including those in the immune tolerant phase, have an increased risk of either advanced liver disease or HCC before reaching the fifth decade of life. In fact, a small prospective study of persons whose average age was 30 years, who were HBeAg-positive and remained so for 5 years, had no or minimal liver disease on biopsy and no significant change on follow-up biopsy.[47]

Unlike hepatitis C virus (HCV) infection, where the viral genotype has little if any influence on the natural history but does predict treatment response, in HBV, genotype has a profound effect on clinical outcome, but with the exception of interferon, has little effect on treatment outcome.[48] There are 8 HBV genotypes that differ by more than 8% in HBV sequence from each other. In addition there are multiple subgenotypes that differ by between 4% and 8%. **Table 4** shows the geographic distribution of the HBV genotypes and subgenotypes identified to date and their HBV-related disease associations. In the United States, genotypes A2 and D are found in persons of European and Middle Eastern descent and genotypes B and C in those of Asian descent.[49] What is important to note is that genotype C appears to be the most deadly of all HBV genotypes. It is associated with high rates of HCC and cirrhosis in middle-aged and older persons beginning in the fifth decade of life and continuing on thereafter. In addition, a large population-based study from Alaska where 5 HBV genotypes are found has shown that the mean age of seroconversion from HBeAg to anti-HBe is younger than 20 for genotypes A, B, D, and F but 47 years for genotype C.[20] This would imply that those infected with genotype C would have, on the average, more years of infection with high viral loads of HBV and may partially explain why the risk of HCC and cirrhosis is so high in persons infected with genotype C. HBV genotype F also has been found to also be associated with a high risk of HCC, especially in persons younger than 30.[50] In Africa, genotype A1 and probably genotypes A3 and E are associated with high rates of HCC, especially for A1 in younger males who are HBeAg negative and frequently do not have cirrhosis.[51] Aflatoxin could play a role as a cofactor in these parts of the world. Subgenotypes B2 to 5 and 7, found in East and Southeast Asia, have a portion of HBV genotype C recombined into the core region of the virus, whereas subgenotypes B1 found in Japan and B6 found in the Arctic, do not have this recombination.[52] In comparative studies, persons infected with genotypes B2 to 5 are, on average, at an older age when HBeAg seroconversion occurs and have an onset of HCC a decade earlier than genotype B1.[53] B6, which is more similar to B1, has not been found to be associated with any instances of HCC or cirrhosis in the Arctic.[54] However, the median age of the population infected is in the fifth decade of life and if this subgenotype behaves more like B1, serious complication would not be expected until the seventh to eighth decades of life. HBV genotype D has been associated with HBeAg-negative active liver disease in which a mutation called pre-core mutant, which takes place at codon 1896, is frequently found.[55] However, it may still be that most persons infected with genotype D seroconvert to anti-HBe and remain in the inactive HBV phase.[22,23] Very little information on the association of HBV genotypes G and H with adverse liver events are available.[48] HBV genotype testing is commercially available but subtypes are not delineated when this testing is performed. However, until we know more about the specific HBV genotype/subtype relationships to disease outcome, this costly test has limited utility.

Two important mutations in the HBV virus have been associated with outcome, the basal core promoter (BCP) mutation and the pre-core (PC) mutation (**Table 5**). The BCP mutation is a double substitution, A1762T, G1764A, in the basal core region of HBV. It has clearly been associated with an increased risk of HCC and cirrhosis in multiple studies, both cross-sectional and prospective.[49,56] For example, in the REVEAL-HBV study discussed previously, the annual incidence of HCC in those with the BCP mutation present versus those with no BCP mutation was 1149 versus 359 per 100,000.[56] The PC mutation is not found in all HBV genotypes, especially genotype A2.[57,58] This mutation typically appears near the time of HBeAg seroconversion. The mutation results in an amino acid change that creates stop codon at site 1846 on the HBV genome so that the virus can transcribe hepatitis B core protein but not HBeAg. If the predominate circulating strain in an individual is the PC strain, then the person may be HBeAg-negative/anti-HBe-positive and have high levels of HBV DNA.[58] Although more common in persons with active liver inflammation, this mutation occurs frequently in persons who have inactive hepatitis also. Many factors may play a role in whether an individual has HBeAg-negative immune active disease including the proportion of the HBV quasispecies with PC mutation plus the strength of

Table 5
Viral factors associated with increased risk of development of hepatocellular carcinoma (HCC) and/or cirrhosis in persons with chronic hepatitis B virus infection

	Increased Risk of HCC	Increased Risk of Cirrhosis
HBV genotype		
Genotype C	3+	2+
Genotype F	2+	no evidence to date
HBV DNA >20,000 IU/mL in persons >40 years	3+	3+
BCP mutation	3+	+
Co-infecting viruses		
HBV/HIV	+	2+
HBV/HCV	3+	2+
HBV/HDV	+	3+

Abbreviations: BCP, basal core promoter; HBV, hepatitis B virus; HCV, hepatitis C virus; HDV, hepatitis D virus; HIV, human immunodeficiency virus.

the immune response against HBV. A recent analysis of the role of PC in the prospective population-based REVEAL-HBV study showed the opposite of what was found in cross-sectional clinic-based studies: that the presence of the PC mutation decreased the annual subsequent incident of HCC (269 per 100,000) and absence increased it (996 per 100,000).[56] Thus, although there is strong evidence that BCP increases the risk of HCC and cirrhosis, the evidence for PC is shaky. Although both tests for PC and PCP mutations are commercially available, it is premature for clinicians to place patients on antiviral therapy based on mutational profile.

OTHER VIRAL CO-INFECTIONS

Patients with HBV who are co-infected with human immunodeficiency virus (HIV), hepatitis C virus (HCV), or hepatitis D virus (HDV) are at an increased risk of developing adverse outcomes to chronic HBV infection. Co-infection with HIV virus is found in between 6% and 15% of persons with HBV (see **Table 5**). The highest prevalence of HIV co-infection is found in sub-Sahara Africa, where the prevalence has been found to be more than 15% in some regions.[59] Although the co-presence of HBV does not appear to affect HIV progression, HIV infection has a profound effect on the outcome of HBV infection. Persons with these two concurrent infections have higher levels on average of HBV DNA and remain HBeAg-positive longer than persons with HBV mono-infection.[60] Furthermore, in HBV/HIV co-infected individuals with low CD4 counts who are given highly active anti-retroviral therapy (HAART) and have reconstitution of their immune system as evidenced by a rise in CD4 counts, flares of hepatitis B are not uncommon and may be misinterpreted as being attributable to drug toxicity.[60,61] Most importantly, persons with HBV/HIV co-infection have been shown to have a high risk of liver-related mortality if only their HIV infection is treated.[62]

The danger of increasing rates of liver-related mortality in HIV-infected persons with HBV co-infection is greatest in sub-Sahara Africa and other countries where HIV screening and treatment programs sponsored by the President's Emergency Program for AIDS Relief (PEPFAR) and the Global AIDS Program (GAP) operate.[63] Currently in these areas, persons identified with HIV are not screened for HBV and those needing HIV treatment are given a cocktail of 3 HAART medications, of which lamivudine is the only one active against HBV. As a result, as many as 90% of HBV/HIV co-infected persons could develop resistant strains of HBV within 3 to 4 years of starting therapy. Over the ensuing decade, the risk of increasing rates of liver-related death caused by HBV in persons whose HIV is under good control is a real threat.[62,64] Fortunately, the World Health Organization (WHO) and GAP in 2010 have recommended changing the treatment paradigm for HBV/HIV co-infected persons by alternatively treating them with a combination that includes tenofovir plus either emtricitabine or lamivudine as part of their HAART regimen. However, it will be a massive undertaking to screen all persons worldwide on HAART for HBsAg to determine which persons are co-infected and evaluate whether a change in their HAART is necessary. However, beginning to screen all newly identified HIV-positive persons for HBsAg and including adequate coverage of HBV in those co-infected would be a good start. Finally, it is important to remember that persons with HIV infection who have low CD4 counts and are immunosuppressed may have high levels of HBV DNA and be HBsAg-negative but only anti-HBc positive.[60] Therefore, it is important to screen HIV-infected persons who are HBsAg-negative but anti-HBc-positive for HBV DNA.

Worldwide, up to 15% of persons with HBV infection are also infected with HCV.[65] The highest risk of HIV/HCV co-infection in developed nations occurs among injecting drug users.[59] However, in the emerging countries, HCV infection is usually caused by breaks in sterile technique from injections, including immunizations and medical procedures.[66] In HBV/HCV co-infected persons, either virus can become the dominant organism; most often HCV assumes that role and suppression of HBV DNA levels can occur.[67] In persons with chronic HBV, acute HCV infection can result in severe or fulminant hepatitis.[68] Long-term infection with both HBV and HCV puts those persons at a higher risk of developing HCC in the future than persons with either HBV or HCV mono-infection.[69]

Hepatitis Delta virus (HDV) is the only known satellite virus that infects humans. Satellite viruses are usually found in plants and require the co-presence of another virus to infect their host. In humans, HDV is dependent on HBV to produce its envelope protein.[70] The HDV RNA genome is only 0.8 Kb and encodes for only one protein, HD-Ag. HBsAg is used as its surface protein allowing the virus to attach to hepatocytes.[70] There are 2 scenarios for HDV infection in humans. HDV co-infection occurs when a person naïve for either virus is infected with both HBV and HDV.[71] This can result in fulminant hepatitis and even death, but in those who recover, more than 90% are immune to both HBV and HDV. In contrast, when HDV superinfection occurs in a person who is already chronically infected with HBV, not only is fulminant hepatitis risk increased but more than 90% of those persons end up chronically infected with both viruses. There are 8 major genotypes of HDV worldwide, differing from each other in nucleotide sequence by as much as 40%.[72] Like HBV, the pathology of HDV differs by HDV genotype. HDV genotype I is found worldwide and is the most common genotype in the United States and Europe. In southern Europe, HBV/HDV co-infection has been found to be associated with a high rate of cirrhosis over time.[73] Genotypes II and IV are found in East Asia and appear to be milder than genotype I.[72] Genotype III is found in the Amazon Delta and is associated with fulminant hepatitis in persons with acute HBV/HDV co-infection, especially when co-infection occurs with HBV genotype F.[74,75] Little is known about the pathogenicity of the other 4 genotypes of HDV.

CHANGING THE NATURAL HISTORY OF CHRONIC HEPATITIS B INFECTION

With the advent of antiviral agents directed against HBV, discussed in another article in this edition of *Clinics of Liver Disease*, the potential to change the natural history of HBV is promising. Already, it has been shown that hepatitis B vaccination can reduce the incidence of HCC in children and prevent HBV infection, thus preventing HBV-related cirrhosis.[76] In addition, clearly treatment of persons with advanced compensated fibrosis and cirrhosis can decrease the incidence of hepatic decompensation, liver-related death, and HCC.[77] Practice guidelines developed by the 3 major liver societies, the American Association for the Study of Liver Diseases (AASLD), the Asian Pacific Association for the Study of the Liver (APASL), and the European Association for the Study of the Liver (EASL), all recommend treatment for those found to have moderate hepatic inflammation or fibrosis, with the reasonable assumption that many of these patients might progress to cirrhosis, despite the lack of evidence, as careful population-based epidemiologic studies to determine if this is the case have not been performed. In developed countries, most persons with chronic HBV, who are immigrants born in endemic countries, have not been detected and are unaware of their infection.[59] The Institute of Medicine came out with a report in January 2010 outlining the problems and barriers that exist to identify, manage, treat, and prevent chronic HBV in the United States, and has made strong recommendations to the US government on how these deficiencies can be improved.[78] Implementation of these recommendations could have a dramatic impact on the natural history of HBV in persons in the United States. The situation in the developing world is not as promising. Currently only a handful of small programs to detect and treat HBV are being conducted in Africa, although more detection and treatment programs are operating in Asia. Programs for hepatitis B immunization of infants are operational in 169 (88%) of the 191 member states of WHO.[79] However, it will take approximately 40 years after implementation of universal newborn/infant immunization to impact the natural history of HBV in persons living in endemic countries, because the incidence of HCC and cirrhosis really do not begin to rise substantially until persons have reached their late 30s and early 40s (see **Fig. 2**). Thus, unless organized programs similar to the PEPFAR program for HIV are funded and established, a dramatic drop in HBV-related liver disease will not be seen for several decades.

In conclusion, the natural history of HBV is complicated and nonlinear. Many infected persons go from a state of high viral load and no or minimal liver disease to one of active liver inflammation followed by a phase of low viral load and inactive liver disease. However, some persons can revert back from inactive to active disease at any time. Thus, persons with chronic HBV must have lifelong, regular monitoring to access disease activity and identify any period where antiviral intervention might be needed. In addition, persons with the highest risk factors for developing HCC, males older than 40, females older than 50, persons with cirrhosis, and those with a family history of HCC should be screened with ultrasound every 6 months as outlined by established practice guidelines, as well as perhaps α-fetoprotein.[30] More population-based natural history studies, such as the REVEAL-HBV study, are needed to identify other characteristics and viral markers that are risk factors for predicting adverse outcome. These markers would include the role of viral genotypes and subtypes that have yet to be studied, specific viral mutations besides BCP, and host immunologic and genetic features that predict outcome, as well as better serologic and radiographic markers that can more accurately identify the stage of liver pathology and fibrosis to allow for more precise timing of antiviral therapy in those who might benefit the most.

REFERENCES

1. Lavanchy D. Hepatitis B virus epidemiology, disease burden, treatment, and current and emerging prevention and control measures. J Viral Hepat 2004; 11(2):97–107.

2. McMahon BJ. The natural history of chronic hepatitis B virus infection. Hepatology 2009;49(5):S45–55.
3. Beasley RP, Hwang LY, Lee GC, et al. Prevention of perinatally transmitted hepatitis B virus infections with hepatitis B virus infections with hepatitis B immune globulin and hepatitis B vaccine. Lancet 1983;2(8359):1099–102.
4. Mast EE, Margolis HS, Fiore AE, et al. A comprehensive immunization strategy to eliminate transmission of hepatitis B virus infection in the United States: recommendations of the Advisory Committee on Immunization Practices (ACIP) part 1: immunization of infants, children, and adolescents. MMWR Recomm Rep 2005;54(RR-16):1–31.
5. Coursaget P, Yvonnet B, Chotard J, et al. Age- and sex-related study of hepatitis B virus chronic carrier state in infants from an endemic area (Senegal). J Med Virol 1987;22(1):1–5.
6. Beasley RP, Hwang LY, Lin CC, et al. Incidence of hepatitis B virus infections in preschool children in Taiwan. J Infect Dis 1982;146(2):198–204.
7. McMahon BJ, Alward WL, Hall DB, et al. Acute hepatitis B virus infection: relation of age to the clinical expression of disease and subsequent development of the carrier state. J Infect Dis 1985;151(4):599–603.
8. Beasley RP. Hepatitis B virus. The major etiology of hepatocellular carcinoma. Cancer 1988;61(10):1942–56.
9. McMahon BJ, Holck P, Bulkow L, et al. Serologic and clinical outcomes 1536 Alaska Natives chronically infected with hepatitis B virus. Ann Intern Med 2001;135:759–68.
10. Di Marco V, Lo Iacono O, Camma C, et al. The long-term course of chronic hepatitis B. Hepatology 1999;30(1):257–64.
11. Fattovich G, Brollo L, Giustina G, et al. Natural history and prognostic factors for chronic hepatitis type B. Gut 1991;32(3):294–8.
12. Fattovich G, Olivari N, Pasino M, et al. Long-term outcome of chronic hepatitis B in Caucasian patients: mortality after 25 years. Gut 2008;57(1):84–90.
13. Yu MW, Hsu FC, Sheen IS, et al. Prospective study of hepatocellular carcinoma and liver cirrhosis in asymptomatic chronic hepatitis B virus carriers. Am J Epidemiol 1997;145(11):1039–47.
14. Liaw YF, Tai DI, Chu CM, et al. The development of cirrhosis in patients with chronic type-B hepatitis—a prospective-study. Hepatology 1988;8(3):493–6.
15. de Jongh FE, Janssen HL, de Man RA, et al. Survival and prognostic indicators in hepatitis B surface antigen-positive cirrhosis of the liver [see comments]. Gastroenterology 1992;103(5):1630–5.
16. Fattovich G, Giustina G, Schalm SW, et al. Occurrence of hepatocellular carcinoma and decompensation in western European patients with cirrhosis type B. The EUROHEP Study Group on Hepatitis B Virus and Cirrhosis. Hepatology 1995;21(1):77–82.
17. Realdi G, Fattovich G, Hadziyannis S, et al. Survival and prognostic factors in 366 patients with compensated cirrhosis type B: a multicenter study. The Investigators of the European Concerted Action on Viral Hepatitis (EUROHEP). J Hepatol 1994;21(4):656–66.
18. Hoofnagle JH, Doo E, Liang TJ, et al. Management of hepatitis B: summary of a clinical research workshop. Hepatology 2007;45(4):1056–75.
19. Sorrell MF, Belongia EA, Costa J, et al. National Institutes of Health consensus development conference statement: management of hepatitis B. Hepatology 2009;49(5):S4–12.
20. Livingston SE, Simonetti JP, Bulkow LR, et al. Clearance of hepatitis B e antigen in patients with chronic hepatitis B and genotypes A, B, C, D, and F. Gastroenterology 2007;133:1452–7.

21. Verling JM. The immunology of hepatitis B. Clin Liver Dis 2007;11:727–59.
22. Zacharakis GH, Koskinas J, Kotsiou S, et al. Natural history of chronic HBV infection: a cohort with up to 12 years follow-up in North Greece (part of the Interreg I-II/EC-Project). J Med Virol 2005;77:173–9.
23. de Franchis R, Meucci G, Vecchi M, et al. The natural-history of asymptomatic hepatitis-B surface-antigen carriers. Ann Intern Med 1993;118(3):191–4.
24. Ahn SH, Park YN, Park JY, et al. Long-term clinical and histological outcomes in patients with spontaneous hepatitis B surface antigen seroclearance. J Hepatol 2005;42(2):188–94.
25. Chu CM, Liaw YF. HBsAg seroclearance in asymptomatic carriers of high endemic areas: appreciably high rates during a long-term follow-up. Hepatology 2007;45(5):1187–92.
26. Simonetti J, Bulkow L, McMahon BJ, et al. Clearance of hepatitis B surface antigen and risk of hepatocellular carcinoma in a cohort chronically infected with hepatitis B virus. Hepatology 2010;51:1531–7.
27. Chen YC, Sheen IS, Chu CM, et al. Prognosis following spontaneous HBsAg seroclearance in chronic hepatitis B patients with or without concurrent infection. Gastroenterology 2002;123(4):1084–9.
28. Huo TI, Wu JC, Lee PC, et al. Sero-clearance of hepatitis B surface antigen in chronic carriers does not necessarily imply a good prognosis [see comments]. Hepatology 1998;28(1):231–6.
29. Yuen MF, Wong DKH, Fung J, et al. HBsAg seroclearance in chronic hepatitis B in Asian patients: replicative level and risk of hepatocellular carcinoma. Gastroenterology 2008;135(4):1192–9.
30. Bruix J, Sherman M. Management of hepatocellular carcinoma. Hepatology 2005;42(5):1208–36.
31. Goldstein ST, Zhou FJ, Hadler SC, et al. A mathematical model to estimate global hepatitis B disease burden and vaccination impact. Int J Epidemiol 2005;34(6):1329–39.
32. McMahon BJ, Bulkow L, Harpster A, et al. Screening for hepatocellular carcinoma in Alaska Natives infected with chronic hepatitis B: a 16-year population-based study. Hepatology 2000;32:842–6.
33. Alberts SR, Lanier AP, McMahon BJ, et al. Clustering of hepatocellular-carcinoma in Alaska Native families. Genet Epidemiol 1991;8(2):127–39.
34. Hainaut P, Boyle P. Curbing the liver cancer epidemic in Africa. Lancet 2008;371(9610):367–8.
35. Kirk GD, Bah E, Montesano R. Molecular epidemiology of human liver cancer: insights into etiology, pathogenesis and prevention from The Gambia, West Africa. Carcinogenesis 2006;27(10):2070–82.
36. Livingston SE, Deubner H, McMahon BJ, et al. Steatosis and hepatitis C in an Alaska Native/American Indian population. Int J Circumpolar Health 2006;65(3):253–60.
37. Wang CS, Yao WJ, Chang TT, et al. The impact of type 2 diabetes on the development of hepatocellular carcinoma in different viral hepatitis statuses. Cancer Epidemiol Biomarkers Prev 2009;18(7):2054–60.
38. Peng DD, Han Y, Ding HG, et al. Hepatic steatosis in chronic hepatitis B patients is associated with metabolic factors more than viral factors. J Gastroenterol Hepatol 2008;23(7):1082–8.
39. Yun JW, Cho YK, Park JH, et al. Hepatic steatosis and fibrosis in young men with treatment-naive chronic hepatitis B. Liver Int 2009;29(6):878–83.

40. Minakari M, Molaei M, Shalmani HM, et al. Liver steatosis in patients with chronic hepatitis B infection: host and viral risk factors. Eur J Gastroenterol Hepatol 2009; 21(5):512–6.
41. Freedman ND, Everhart JE, Lindsay KL, et al. Coffee intake is associated with lower rates of liver disease progression in chronic hepatitis C. Hepatology 2009;50(5):1360–9.
42. Chen CJ, Yang HI, Su J, et al. Risk of hepatocellular carcinoma across a biological gradient of serum hepatitis B virus DNA level. JAMA 2006;295(1):65–73.
43. Harris RA, Chen G, Lin WY, et al. Spontaneous clearance of high-titer serum HBV DNA and risk of hepatocellular carcinoma in a Chinese population. Cancer Causes Control 2003;14(10):995–1000.
44. Yang HI, Lu SN, Liaw YF, et al. Hepatitis B e antigen and the risk of hepatocellular carcinoma. N Engl J Med 2002;347(3):168–74.
45. Yu MW, Yeh SH, Chen PJ, et al. Hepatitis B virus genotype and DNA level and hepatocellular carcinoma: a prospective study in men. J Natl Cancer Inst 2005; 97(4):265–72.
46. Lok ASF, McMahon BJ. Chronic hepatitis B: update 2009. Hepatology 2009;50(3): 661–2.
47. Hui CK, Leung N, Yuen ST, et al. Natural history and disease progression in Chinese chronic hepatitis B patients in immune-tolerant phase. Hepatology 2007;46(2):395–401.
48. McMahon BJ. The influence of hepatitis B virus genotype and subgenotype on the natural history of chronic hepatitis B. Hepatol Int 2009;3(2):334–42.
49. Chu CJ, Keeffe EB, Han SH, et al. Hepatitis B virus genotypes in the United States: results of a nationwide study. Gastroenterology 2003; 125(2):444–51.
50. Livingston SE, Simonetti JP, McMahon BJ, et al. Hepatitis B virus genotypes in Alaska native people with hepatocellular carcinoma: preponderance of genotype F. J Infect Dis 2007;195(1):5–11.
51. Kramvis A, Kew MC, Bukofzer S. Hepatitis B virus precore mutants in serum and liver of Southern African blacks with hepatocellular carcinoma. J Hepatol 1998; 28(1):132–41.
52. Saugauchi F, Orito E, Ichida T, et al. Epidemiologic and virologic characteristics of hepatitis B virus genotype B having the recombination with genotype C. Gastroenterology 2003;124:925–32.
53. Kao JH. Hepatitis B virus genotypes and hepatocellular carcinoma in Taiwan. Intervirology 2003;46(6):400–7.
54. Sakamoto T, Tanaka Y, Simonetti J, et al. Classification of hepatitis B virus genotype B into 2 major types based on characterization of a novel subgenotype in Arctic indigenous populations. J Infect Dis 2007;196:1487–92.
55. Hadziyannis SJ, Vassilopoulos D. Hepatitis B e antigen-negative chronic hepatitis B. Hepatology 2001;34(4):617–24.
56. Yang HI, Yeh SH, Chen PJ, et al. Associations between hepatitis B virus genotype and mutants and the risk of hepatocellular carcinoma. J Natl Cancer Inst 2008; 100(16):1134–43.
57. Grandjacques C, Pradat P, Stuyver L, et al. Rapid detection of genotypes and mutations in the pre-core promoter and the pre-core region of hepatitis B virus genome: correlation with viral persistence and disease severity. J Hepatol 2000;33(3):430–9.
58. Naoumov NV, Schneider R, Grotzinger T, et al. Precore mutant hepatitis-B virus infection and liver disease. Gastroenterology 1992;102(2):538–43.

59. Weinbaum CM, Mast EE, Ward JW. Recommendations for identification and public health management of persons with chronic hepatitis B virus infection. Hepatology 2009;49(5):S35–44.

60. Soriano V, Puoti M, Bonacini M, et al. Care of patients with chronic hepatitis B and HIV co-infection: recommendations from an HIV-HBV International Panel. AIDS 2005;19(3):221–40.

61. Hoffmann CJ, Charalambous S, Martin DJ, et al. Hepatitis B virus infection and response to antiretroviral therapy (ART) in a South African ART program. Clin Infect Dis 2008;47(11):1479–85.

62. Thio CL, Seaberg EC, Skolasky R, et al. HIV-1, hepatitis B virus, and risk of liver-related mortality in the Multicenter Cohort Study (MACS). Lancet 2002;360(9349): 1921–6.

63. Bendavid E, Bhattacharya J. The president's emergency plan for AIDS relief in Africa: an evaluation of outcomes. Ann Intern Med 2009;150(10):688–95.

64. Modi AA, Feld JJ. Viral hepatitis and HIV in Africa. AIDS Rev 2007;9(1):25–39.

65. Strader DB. Understudied populations with hepatitis C. Hepatology 2002;36(5 Suppl 1):S226–36.

66. Lavanchy D. The global burden of hepatitis C. Liver Int 2009;29:74–81.

67. Liaw YF, Tsai SL, Chang JJ, et al. Displacement of hepatitis B virus by hepatitis C virus as the cause of continuing chronic hepatitis. Gastroenterology 1994;106(4): 1048–53.

68. Chu CM, Yeh CT, Liaw YF. Fulminant hepatic failure in acute hepatitis C: increased risk in chronic carriers of hepatitis B virus. Gut 1999;45(4):613–7.

69. Donato F, Boffetta P, Puoti M. A meta-analysis of epidemiological studies on the combined effect of hepatitis B and C virus infections in causing hepatocellular carcinoma. Int J Cancer 1998;75(3):347–54.

70. Taylor JM. Hepatitis delta virus. Virology 2006;344(1):71–6.

71. Hadziyannis SJ. Hepatitis D. Clin Liver Dis 1999;3:309–25.

72. Rizzetto M. Hepatitis D: thirty years after. J Hepatol 2009;50(5):1043–50.

73. Fattovich G, Giustina G, Christensen E, et al. Influence of hepatitis delta virus infection on morbidity and mortality in compensated cirrhosis type B. The European Concerted Action on Viral Hepatitis (Eurohep). Gut 2000;46(3):420–6.

74. Nakano T, Shapiro CN, Hadler SC, et al. Characterization of hepatitis D virus genotype III among Yucpa Indians in Venezuela. J Gen Virol 2001;82:2183–9.

75. Hadler SC, Demonzon M, Ponzetto A, et al. Delta virus-infection and severe hepatitis—an epidemic in the Yucpa Indians of Venezuela. Ann Intern Med 1984; 100(3):339–44.

76. Chang MH, Chen CJ, Lai MS, et al. Universal hepatitis B vaccination in Taiwan and the incidence of hepatocellular carcinoma in children. N Engl J Med 1997; 336(26):1855–9.

77. Liaw YF, Sung JJ, Chow WC, et al. Lamivudine for patients with chronic hepatitis B and advanced liver disease. N Engl J Med 2004;351(15):1521–31.

78. Beasley RP, Alter HJ, Brandeau ML, et al. Institute of Medicine: Hepatitis and Liver Cancer: A National Strategy for Prevention and Control of Hepatitis B and C. In: Colvin HM, Mitchell AE, editors. Washington, DC: National Academies Press; 2010. p. 1–232.

79. Centers for Disease Control and Prevention. Implementation of newborn hepatitis B vaccination—worldwide, 2006. MMWR Morb Mortal Wkly Rep 2008;57(46): 1249–52.

Hepatitis B Virology for Clinicians

Edward C. Doo, MD[a], Marc G. Ghany, MD, MHSc[b],*

KEYWORDS

• Hepatitis B virus • Polymerase • Antiviral Therapy • cccDNA

The expanding knowledge on the hepatitis B virus (HBV) life cycle has improved the understanding of the human disease caused by this virus and led to the development of better treatments. It is important for the clinician taking care of patients with chronic hepatitis B to have a basic understanding of the molecular events involved in the HBV life cycle, so that they can better appreciate the natural history and atypical presentations of the disease and can develop individual management plans based on readily available virologic tests. This article serves to introduce the clinically relevant aspects of the HBV life cycle as they pertain to patient management.

VIROLOGY
The Virus

The human HBV is a member of the Hepadnaviridae family.[1] Humans and higher-order primates are the only known hosts for human HBV. Other HBVs related to the human virus specifically infect hosts such as the ground squirrels, woodchucks, Peking ducks, and herons and serve as models of disease caused by human HBV.[1]

As visualized by electron microscopy, serum from patients with acute and chronic HBV infection exhibit 3 types of particles.[2] The largest particle, a 42-nm spherical structure with a lipid bilayer, is referred to as the Dane particle and represents the intact virion. The outer lipid bilayer derived from host hepatocytes is studded with the hepatitis B surface antigen (HBsAg) and surrounds an inner nucleocapsid with an icosahedral structure composed of hepatitis B core antigen

The authors received no commercial funding for this work.

Financial support: This research was supported by the Intramural Research Program of the National Institutes of Health, Nutrition, National Institute of Diabetes and Digestive and Kidney Diseases.

[a] Liver Diseases Research Branch, Division of Digestive Diseases and Nutrition, National Institute of Diabetes and Digestive and Kidney Diseases, National Institutes of Health, Two Democracy Plaza, Room 651, MSC 5450, 6707 Democracy Boulevard, Bethesda, MD 20892-5450, USA

[b] Liver Diseases Branch, National Institute of Diabetes and Digestive and Kidney Diseases, National Institutes of Health, Building 10 Room 9B-16, 10 Center Drive, MSC 1800, Bethesda, MD 20892-1800, USA

* Corresponding author.

E-mail address: Marcg@intra.niddk.nih.gov

Clin Liver Dis 14 (2010) 397–408

doi:10.1016/j.cld.2010.05.001

1089-3261/10/$ – see front matter © 2010 Published by Elsevier Inc.

liver.theclinics.com

(HBcAg). The HBV genome and the viral polymerase reside within the nucleocapsid. The other 2 particles visualized by electron microscopy appear either as small spherical particles or as filaments approximately 20 to 22 nm in size. These particles are devoid of any HBV genome and are composed of just host lipids and HBsAg; therefore, these particles are noninfectious.[3] The subvirion particles are usually present in significant excess than the Dane particles, but why they are produced in such great numbers is unknown. It has been speculated that these noninfectious particles and filaments may serve as a decoy for the immune system and aid in the establishment of chronic infection. All 3 particles have a common antigen on their surface termed the HBsAg. Detection of HBsAg is the basis of the serologic assay for the diagnosis of chronic hepatitis B.

Genomic Organization

HBV is one of the smallest DNA viruses to infect humans. The HBV genome is a partially double-stranded circular DNA of approximately 3.2 kb in length.[1,4] A unique feature of the genome is that the 2 DNA strands are asymmetric.[4] The minus strand is genome length, whereas the complimentary positive strand is of variable length. There are 4 open reading frames (core [C], polymerase [P], surface [S], and X) that partially overlap because of the compact nature of the genome (**Fig. 1**). Four viral messenger RNAs (mRNAs) are generated from the viral genome.[1,4] The C and S genes have a single open reading frame with multiple in-frame start codons that give rise to related but functionally different gene products. The mRNAs are designated by their lengths as a 3.5-kb pregenomic mRNA, a 2.4-kb large surface mRNA, a 2.1-kb middle and small surface mRNA, and a 0.7-kb X mRNA.[1,4] The 3.5-kb length mRNA actually exists as 2 subspecies: a slightly longer precore-core 3.5-kb mRNA and a shorter pregenomic 3.5-kb mRNA. The precore-core mRNA yields the precore –core protein, which undergoes posttranslational modification to give rise to the secretory hepatitis B e antigen (HBeAg) protein, whereas the pregenomic mRNA gives rise to the core and polymerase proteins and also serves as the template for replication of the virus. The biologic function of the HBeAg remains obscure. HBeAg is not required for viral replication but seems to be necessary for the establishment of chronic infection by acting as a tolerogen.[5] Clinically, detection of HBeAg correlates with high-level viremia.[6] Reduction in HBeAg level either spontaneously or during treatment is an important milestone in the natural history of the disease because it serves to indicate a transition from a high to a low viral replicative state.[7] The S gene gives rise to 2 mRNA transcripts: a 2.4-kb large surface mRNA and a 2.1-kb middle and small surface mRNA. These 2 transcripts yield the 3 surface antigen proteins: large, middle, and small.[1,4] All the three HBsAgs share the same carboxy-terminal region. The 0.7-kb X mRNA translates to yield the X protein. The function of the X protein (hepatitis B X antigen) remains incompletely understood, but emerging evidence seems to support a role in productive HBV replication, transcriptional activation, and DNA repair.[8,9]

Viral Life Cycle

The first step of initiating a productive infection involves the attachment of the mature Dane particle to the outer hepatocyte membrane through an unidentified host receptor. Evidence suggests that the large HBsAg plays a role in the attachment process.[10,11] After attachment, the Dane particle is internalized into the cytoplasm and undergoes a series of transformations involving disassembly of the lipid bilayer

Organization of HBV Genome

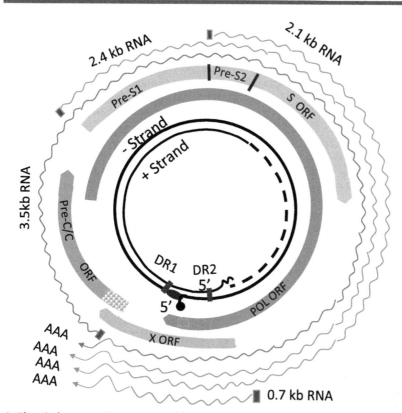

Fig. 1. The viral genome is represented by the inner, black circles. It is a relaxed circular partially double-stranded DNA. The DNA's circularity is maintained by 5'-cohesive ends containing 2 11-nucleotide direct repeats that are important for viral replication. The 2 strands are asymmetric. The minus strand is genome length and is covalently linked at its 5' end to the terminal protein domain of polymerase. The positive strand is of variable length and has a capped oligoribonucleotide on its 5' end. The genome has 4 open reading frames, which overlap due to the compact nature of the genome. These are all encoded by the minus strand and consist of the polymerase, precore/core, pre-S1/pre-S2, s/pre-s, and X. Finally, the outer wavy lines represent 4 viral messenger RNA (mRNA) species. The 3.5-kb pregenomic mRNA is genome length and the other 3 are subgenomic length. All terminate in a poly A tail.

and dissolution of the nucleocapsid.[1,4] The relaxed circular form of the viral DNA is delivered to the nucleus where host and viral polymerases repair the partially double-stranded DNA to form the covalently closed circular DNA (cccDNA). The conversion of the relaxed circular DNA to a cccDNA involves the extension of the positive strand to full length, removal of the relaxed circular DNA's terminal modifications, and covalent ligation of the DNA ends.[1,4,12,13] The cccDNA serves as the template for transcription of all the viral mRNAs.

The HBV mRNAs are then transported into the cytoplasm where translation of the viral proteins, self-assembly of core protein molecules into nucleocapsids, and progeny genome replication occurs.[1,4] Replication requires encapsidation of the pre-genomic RNA by the core particle. This process is initiated by the coordinated binding of the viral polymerase to a secondary stem-loop structure, termed epsilon, on the pregenomic 3.5-kb mRNA, which triggers encapsidation by the core protein to form the viral nucleocapsid.[14]

After binding of the HBV polymerase to epsilon on the pregenomic mRNA, the poly-merase then serves as a protein primer to initiate negative-strand DNA synthesis. Elongation of a newly synthesized negative DNA strand subsequently proceeds with the pregenomic 3.5-kb mRNA serving as the template. After completion of the negative-strand DNA synthesis, the 3.5-kb mRNA template is degraded by the viral ribonuclease (RNase) H domain of the polymerase. Thereafter, the partially duplex HBV genome is synthesized using the newly synthesized negative strand as the template. The positive-strand synthesis is rarely complete, and thus the variable length of the positive strand in the HBV virion. Finally, the partially duplex HBV genome circularizes to assume the partially double-stranded, relaxed circular conformation within the nucleocapsid.[1,4] Although HBV replicates via an RNA intermediate step, integration of the HBV DNA into the host DNA is not a requirement for replication as opposed to human immunodeficiency virus (HIV) in which the integration is essential for the life cycle.

Once the viral genome synthesis is completed, the immature viral nucleocapsid has 2 fates: it can acquire a lipid membrane with the HBsAg proteins in the endoplasmic reticulum to form mature Dane particles that are secreted from the hepatocyte or it can be transported back to the nucleus to replenish the pool of cccDNA.

The cccDNA

The cccDNA is central to the durability of HBV infection. It resides in the nucleus of infected hepatocytes as a stable, nonintegrated episomal DNA.[15] The cccDNA assumes a supercoiled conformation that is reminiscent of a chromosomal structure complete with histone binding.[16,17] The number of cccDNA molecules in each infected hepatocyte nucleus varies, ranging from 1 to 50 per cell nuclei.[16,17] Unlike the hepa-tocyte chromosome, the cccDNA is not replicated by the host DNA replication machinery. Rather, maintenance of cccDNA is through an intracellular recycling pathway whereby newly synthesized but immature nucleocapsids are recycled from the cytoplasm to the nucleus to replenish the cccDNA level.[18] Factors that regulate the number of cccDNA molecules in each nucleus remain incompletely understood. Immunologic, virologic, and epigenetic factors, including transcription factors, have been suggested to regulate cccDNA levels.[15,19]

cccDNA seems to be very stable within the hepatocyte and has been shown to persist after antiviral therapy and even after clearance of HBsAg in both animal and human studies.[20–25] Because cccDNA serves as the template for the viral mRNAs, its stability in hepatocytes means that it can be a constant source of future viral progeny. Thus, cccDNA plays a significant role in reactivation of disease after stop-ping of antiviral treatment, following withdrawal of immunosuppression, in de novo hepatitis B after transplantation of anti-hepatitis B core grafts, and in the development of drug resistance. A particular concern over the use of oral nucleoside or nucleotide analogues is the archiving of resistant mutations in cccDNA, which may contribute to the development of multidrug-resistant viruses. Persistence of cccDNA is a major challenge in successfully eradicating HBV. Two leading mechanisms seem to be important for elimination of cccDNA. The first mechanism is based on a cytolytic mechanism by which infected hepatocytes are killed and replaced by regenerating noninfected hepatocytes.[26,27] The second mechanism is based on a noncytolytic mechanism, whereby antiviral cytokines downregulate HBV gene expression and eliminate HBV from hepatocytes without cell death.[28,29] Evidence exists for both mechanisms.

Given the central role of cccDNA in HBV replication, it is an attractive target for therapeutic intervention. Current treatment strategies have had little effect on cccDNA levels. In particular, nucleoside or nucleotide analogue inhibitors of the HBV polymerase do not have a direct effect on cccDNA. Rather, they indirectly affect cccDNA levels through the abrogation of the intracellular recycling pathway. Several studies have examined the change in cccDNA levels during therapy with currently available nucleoside or nucleotide analogues used as monotherapy and in combination with peginterferon (**Fig. 2**).[21,22,24,30,31] In all cases, with the exception of peginterferon plus adefovir dipivoxil,[30] therapy for 1 year was associated with only modest reduction in cccDNA levels and none resulted in elimination of cccDNA. In contrast, serum HBV-DNA levels decreased by 4.7 to 5.5 $\log_{10}$ and cytoplasmic HBV-DNA levels in the hepatocytes decreased by about 2 $\log_{10}$. Based on currently available treatment data, mathematical modeling has projected that a therapeutic duration of 12 to 14 years would be necessary to achieve eradication of cccDNA from the liver. Recent data identifying cellular factors involved in the regulation of cccDNA may lead to the development of new antiviral therapies.[32,33]

The Polymerase

The HBV polymerase has a central role in the synthesis of new virions. Knowledge of the structure-function relationship of the HBV polymerase has allowed a better understanding of how current nucleoside or nucleotide therapy works and conversely why it fails.[34] The HBV polymerase is a multifunctional protein that is organized into 4 distinct domains beginning with a terminal protein domain at the amino-terminus region followed by a spacer region domain, a reverse transcriptase domain, and ending with an RNase H domain at the carboxy-terminus region. The terminal protein and spacer domains are unique to the HBV polymerase, with no phylogenetically related structures present on other viral polymerases.[35] The terminal

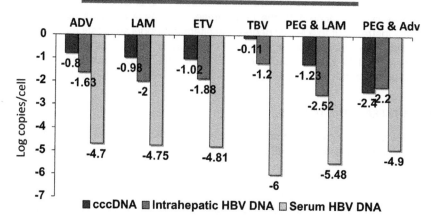

Fig. 2. Comparison of change in cccDNA, intrahepatic, and serum HBV-DNA levels after antiviral therapy for 48 to 52 weeks.

protein domain is absolutely essential for replication of the HBV genome.[36,37] Similar to the replication schemes of other viruses, HBV uses a protein instead of the classic RNA or DNA termini as the primer for initiating DNA synthesis. Specifically, a tyrosine residue within the terminal protein domain acts as a primer and covalently links to the first nucleotide of the nascent negative-strand DNA.[38,39] In contrast, the function of the spacer region is unknown and is dispensable without affecting polymerase function. Unlike the terminal protein and spacer domains, the reverse transcriptase and RNase H domains share sequence motifs with other viral polymerases.[35] The reverse transcriptase domain can be subdivided into 7 subdomains designated A to G.[35] The subdomain C encompasses the DNA polymerization active site of the HBV polymerase and is the site of action for oral nucleoside or nucleotide analogues. The RNase H domain degrades the pregenomic mRNA template after negative-strand synthesis.

The crystal structure of the HBV polymerase has not been resolved. However, based on sequence homology with the HIV-1 reverse transcriptase and on the similar pattern of resistant mutations that occur with antiviral compounds that have both HBV and HIV activity, several predictions about the HBV polymerase can be made. Like other viral polymerases, HBV polymerase also has a right-handed structure with fingers, palm, and thumb regions.[35] The palm region serves as the catalytically active site of the reverse transcriptase domain, where incoming nucleotides are attached to the elongating DNA of a new HBV genome. Structurally, the subdomains A, C, and perhaps D participate directly in nucleotide binding and catalysis.[35] Subdomains B and E are involved with precise positioning of the primer-template complex relative to the incoming nucleotide in the active site and are components of the fingers and thumb regions.[35]

Nucleoside or nucleotide analogues inhibit HBV-DNA synthesis by acting as DNA chain terminators. Structurally, these analogues lack the 3'-hydroxyl group that permits covalent bonding to an incoming nucleotide on the elongating DNA chain. Therefore, after incorporation of the nucleoside or nucleotide analogue into the nascent DNA chain, subsequent nucleotides are unable to covalently bond with the analogue resulting in termination of replication. These analogues are potent inhibitors of HBV replication. However, a major challenge of nucleoside or nucleotide analogue therapy is the development of resistance mutations. Structure-function modeling helps to understand the mechanisms of resistance. In the case of lamivudine, structure-function modeling suggests that HBV polymerase–resistant mutations alter the spatial conformation of the nucleotide-binding pocket by steric hindrance, thus limiting lamivudine access to the polymerase.[40,41] These changes also affect the natural substrate but to a lesser degree. An alternate model suggests that lamivudine may bind to the resistant polymerase but in a manner that is strained relative to the configuration of the wild-type polymerase.[41] In this strained configuration, the position of lamivudine on the replication complex is not suitable for efficient catalysis.

OTHER THERAPEUTIC TARGETS

The widespread problem of drug resistance associated with nucleoside and nucleotide analogues targeting the HBV polymerase has led investigators to explore other targets for drug development. The identification of other targets for antiviral drug development stems from the knowledge gained through the understanding of the basic molecular biology of the HBV life cycle (**Fig. 3**). Stepwise advancements have been made in understanding the virion attachment to the hepatocyte, the assembly of nucleocapsids, and the mature virus and in the science of antisense and short interfering RNAs (siRNAs).

Molecular Targets to Inhibit HBV Replication

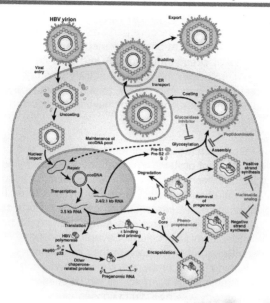

Fig. 3. The small compact genome and the requirement of host cellular enzymes for many stages of the HBV life cycle have been an impediment to antiviral drug development. However, a better understanding of the HBV life cycle has identified several molecular targets and compounds that can disrupt new virion formation. These include viral entry inhibitors, encapsidation inhibitors, and agents that prevent viral assembly and coating. Heteroaryldihydropyrimidines (HAPs) bind to the core particles and lead to their degradation. Another group of compounds that inhibit the encapsidation step are phenylpropenamides. These compounds directly inhibit formation of the nucleocapsid. Antisense RNA and short interfering RNA (siRNA) have been shown to inhibit viral assembly in vitro and in animal models. Glucosidase inhibitors block the glycosylation of surface proteins during the viral assembly step. Recently, pre-S1 derived lipopeptides were shown to be potent inhibitors of HBV entry and may be useful after liver transplantation and perhaps in chronic hepatitis B. (*From* Ghany M, Liang TJ. Drug targets and molecular mechanisms of drug resistance in chronic hepatitis B. Gastroenterology 2007;132:1574–85; with permission.)

Inhibitors of Nucleocapsid Assembly

The HBcAg serves as the structural unit in the assembly of the viral nucleocapsid. As previously discussed, initiation of nucleocapsid formation occurs with the interaction of the HBV polymerase with epsilon on the pregenomic 3.5-kb mRNA, signaling the recruitment of HBcAg. Subsequently, HBcAg units aggregate on the initial complex and through a process of self-assembly lead to nucleocapsid formation. Heteroaryldihydropyrimidines (HAPs) are a class of compounds that have been shown to interfere with the HBcAg self-assembly into nucleocapsids and therefore inhibit HBV replication in a transgenic mouse model.[42] The precise molecular mechanism by which HAPs disrupt nucleocapsid formation is unclear. Some studies suggest that HAPs accelerate nucleocapsid formation but in a disordered fashion.[43–45] The misassembled nucleocapsid is subsequently recognized by the host's unfolded-protein response and is subjected to degradation by cellular proteosomes.[43,44] This approach of inhibiting HBV replication represents a promising direction for drug development.

Another class of compounds with nucleocapsid-assembly inhibitory activity are the phenylpropenamides. One derivative, AT-61, was found to be a potent inhibitor of HBV replication in tissue culture models.[46,47] AT-61 was equally effective at inhibiting both the formation of intracellular immature core particles and the release of virions from hepatocytes. It seems to be active at one of the steps between the synthesis of viral RNA and the packaging of pregenomic mRNA into immature core particles.[46,47] A related compound, AT-130, with more potent activity was reported to block HBV replication at the level of pregenomic mRNA packaging into nucleocapsids.[48] To date, no human studies with these compounds have been reported.

Inhibitors of Viral Assembly

Glycosylation of the HBsAg is a requirement for viral assembly and proper function of the protein.[1] N-glycosylation of proteins is important for proper folding of proteins by mediating interactions between the lectinlike endoplasmic reticulum chaperone proteins, calnexin and calreticulin. However, the N-glycans must first be modified by α-glucosidases to facilitate this interaction. These interactions can be prevented by inhibitors of α-glucosidases, which cause some proteins to be misfolded and retained within the endoplasmic reticulum. Several iminosugar compounds have been shown to have antiviral activity, although their mechanism of action is incompletely understood. An iminosugar compound, N-nonyl-deoxynojirimycin, was shown to inhibit woodchuck hepatitis virus in an animal model of infection.[49] Evidence suggested that the antiviral activity was by a direct consequence of glucosidase inhibition and disruption of virion assembly via a dominant negative effect.[49] However, another related compound N-nonyl-deoxygalactojirimycin (N-nonyl-DGJ), an alkyl derivative of galactose, had no effect on glycoprocessing yet retained anti-HBV activity.[50] This property of N-nonyl-DGJ suggests that it exerted its antiviral action at a point before nucleocapsid envelopment by host membranes and may prevent the proper encapsidation of the HBV pregenomic mRNA.[50] As with any agent that targets a host protein, there is the potential for toxicity, and these agents have been inadequately assessed in humans.

Inhibitors of Viral Entry

The development of the HBV-susceptible cell line HepaRG has facilitated systematic investigations of HBV entry and resulted in the discovery of entry inhibitors derived from viral envelope proteins. Several N-terminal myristoylated or steroylated pre-S1 peptides encompassing the amino acid positions 2 to 47 or 2 to 39 have been shown to block virus infectivity with a 50% inhibitory concentrations ranging from 8 to 300 nM.[51] The postulated mechanism of action is unknown and may be through interaction and inactivation of a cellular receptor or viral protein. At present, the potential role of viral peptide–derived lipoproteins would be primarily preventative and limited to postexposure prophylaxis, prevention of vertical transmission, or graft reinfection after liver transplant. Whether these agents would have any role in patients with chronic infection is currently unknown.

GENETIC APPROACHES

RNA interference is an evolutionary conserved mechanism that uses short RNAs in association with an effector complex referred to as the RNA-induced silencing complex to regulate gene expression in a sequence-specific manner.[52] Two classes of small RNAs mediate this process: microRNAs (miRNAs) and siRNAs.[52] HBV is a promising target for an RNA interference approach because its compact genome lacks significant redundancy. Several approaches have been aimed at using in vitro and animal models with varying results. siRNA sequences targeting most of the subgenomic viral mRNAs have been tested and resulted in ~60% to 80% reduction in protein expression from the targeted gene.[52] Short hairpin RNAs have also been used and possess the advantage of being expressed from plasmids or viral vectors. Results are similar to those obtained with siRNAs. A promising approach may be the use of trimeric miRNA shuttle cassettes, which allows targeting of multiple sequences from a single transcript.

At present, this technology is still nascent with many technical challenges that need to be resolved before it can find widespread human application. The following challenges are common to this therapeutic approach for a multitude of diseases: how to effectively deliver the siRNA or miRNA, how to achieve long-term gene silencing, how to deliver the molecule to the target site of action, and how to deal with the potential for toxicity.

SUMMARY

A comprehensive, detailed understanding of the HBV life cycle and the host-virus interactions has led to the development of successful oral therapy for chronic hepatitis B and the identification of several promising new targets. The development of agents directed toward these targets may lead to new therapies for patients with chronic hepatitis B. With the improved knowledge gained from studying the molecular biology of HBV, novel approaches to inhibition of viral replication are being explored, such as viral entry inhibitors, nucleocapsid inhibitors, and inhibitors of viral assembly. However, the ultimate goal of therapy is to identify strategies to eliminate cccDNA from infected hepatocytes, which would have the potential to be curative and to prevent transmission and could reduce an infected individual's risk for hepatocellular carcinoma. The future seems optimistic for addressing these goals.

REFERENCES

1. Seeger C, Zoulim F, Mason WS. Hepadnaviridae. In: Knipe DM, Roizman B, Howley PM, et al, editors. Fields virology. 5th edition. Philadelphia: Lippincott-Raven Publishers; 2007.
2. Gerber MA, Hadziyannis S, Vissoulis C, et al. Electron microscopy and immunoelectronmicroscopy of cytoplasmic hepatitis B antigen in hepatocytes. Am J Pathol 1974;75:489–502.
3. Gavilanes F, Gonzalez-Ros JM, Peterson DL. Structure of hepatitis B surface antigen. Characterization of the lipid components and their association with the viral proteins. J Biol Chem 1982;257:7770–7.
4. Seeger C, Mason WS. Hepatitis B virus biology. Microbiol Mol Biol Rev 2000;64: 51–68.
5. Milich D, Liang TJ. Exploring the biological basis of hepatitis B e antigen in hepatitis B virus infection. Hepatology 2003;38:1075–86.
6. Perrillo R, Campbell C, Wellinghoff W, et al. The relationship of hepatitis B e antigen, DNA polymerase activity, and titer of hepatitis B surface antigen with ongoing liver injury in chronic hepatitis B virus infection. Am J Gastroenterol 1982;77:445–9.
7. Hoofnagle JH, Dusheiko GM, Seeff LB, et al. Seroconversion from hepatitis B e antigen to antibody in chronic type B hepatitis. Ann Intern Med 1981;94: 744–8.

8. Cross JC, Wen P, Rutter WJ. Transactivation by hepatitis B virus X protein is promiscuous and dependent on mitogen-activated cellular serine/threonine kinases. Proc Natl Acad Sci U S A 1993;90:8078–82.

9. Bouchard MJ, Schneider RJ. The enigmatic X gene of hepatitis B virus. J Virol 2004;78:12725–34.

10. Glebe D, Urban S, Knoop EV, et al. Mapping of the hepatitis B virus attachment site by use of infection-inhibiting preS1 lipopeptides and tupaia hepatocytes. Gastroenterology 2005;129:234–45.

11. Klingmuller U, Schaller H. Hepadnavirus infection requires interaction between the viral pre-S domain and a specific hepatocellular receptor. J Virol 1993;67:7414–22.

12. Kock J, Schlicht HJ. Analysis of the earliest steps of hepadnavirus replication: genome repair after infectious entry into hepatocytes does not depend on viral polymerase activity. J Virol 1993;67:4867–74.

13. Sohn JA, Litwin S, Seeger C. Mechanism for CCC DNA synthesis in hepadnaviruses. PLoS One 2009;4:e8093.

14. Pollack JR, Ganem D. An RNA stem-loop structure directs hepatitis B virus genomic RNA encapsidation. J Virol 1993;67:3254–63.

15. Zoulim F. New insight on hepatitis B virus persistence from the study of intrahepatic viral cccDNA. J Hepatol 2005;42:302–8.

16. Tuttleman JS, Pourcel C, Summers J. Formation of the pool of covalently closed circular viral DNA in hepadnavirus-infected cells. Cell 1986;47:451–60.

17. Newbold JE, Xin H, Tencza M, et al. The covalently closed duplex form of the hepadnavirus genome exists in situ as a heterogeneous population of viral minichromosomes. J Virol 1995;69:3350–7.

18. Wu TT, Coates L, Aldrich CE, et al. In hepatocytes infected with duck hepatitis B virus, the template for viral RNA synthesis is amplified by an intracellular pathway. Virology 1990;175:255–61.

19. Levrero M, Pollicino T, Petersen J, et al. Control of cccDNA function in hepatitis B virus infection. J Hepatol 2009;51:581–92.

20. Mason WS, Cullen J, Moraleda G, et al. Lamivudine therapy of WHV-infected woodchucks. Virology 1998;245:18–32.

21. Yuen MF, Wong DK, Sum SS, et al. Effect of lamivudine therapy on the serum covalently closed-circular (ccc) DNA of chronic hepatitis B infection. Am J Gastroenterol 2005;100:1099–103.

22. Wong DK, Yuen MF, Ngai VW, et al. One-year entecavir or lamivudine therapy results in reduction of hepatitis B virus intrahepatic covalently closed circular DNA levels. Antivir Ther 2006;11:909–16.

23. Bourne EJ, Dienstag JL, Lopez VA, et al. Quantitative analysis of HBV cccDNA from clinical specimens: correlation with clinical and virological response during antiviral therapy. J Viral Hepat 2007;14:55–63.

24. Werle-Lapostolle B, Bowden S, Locarnini S, et al. Persistence of cccDNA during the natural history of chronic hepatitis B and decline during adefovir dipivoxil therapy. Gastroenterology 2004;126:1750–8.

25. Moraleda G, Saputelli J, Aldrich CE, et al. Lack of effect of antiviral therapy in nondividing hepatocyte cultures on the closed circular DNA of woodchuck hepatitis virus. J Virol 1997;71:9392–9.

26. Fourel I, Cullen JM, Saputelli J, et al. Evidence that hepatocyte turnover is required for rapid clearance of duck hepatitis B virus during antiviral therapy of chronically infected ducks. J Virol 1994;68:8321–30.

27. Guo JT, Zhou H, Liu C, et al. Apoptosis and regeneration of hepatocytes during recovery from transient hepadnavirus infections. J Virol 2000;74:1495–505.

28. Thimme R, Wieland S, Steiger C, et al. CD8(+) T cells mediate viral clearance and disease pathogenesis during acute hepatitis B virus infection. J Virol 2003;77:68–76.
29. Guidotti LG, Rochford R, Chung J, et al. Viral clearance without destruction of infected cells during acute HBV infection. Science 1999;284:825–9.
30. Wursthorn K, Lutgehetmann M, Dandri M, et al. Peginterferon alpha-2b plus adefovir induce strong cccDNA decline and HBsAg reduction in patients with chronic hepatitis B. Hepatology 2006;44:675–84.
31. Sung JJ, Wong ML, Bowden S, et al. Intrahepatic hepatitis B virus covalently closed circular DNA can be a predictor of sustained response to therapy. Gastroenterology 2005;128:1890–7.
32. Belloni L, Pollicino T, De Nicola F, et al. Nuclear HBx binds the HBV minichromosome and modifies the epigenetic regulation of cccDNA function. Proc Natl Acad Sci U S A 2009;106:19975–9.
33. Turin F, Borel C, Benchaib M, et al. n-Butyrate, a cell cycle blocker, inhibits early amplification of duck hepatitis B virus covalently closed circular DNA after in vitro infection of duck hepatocytes. J Virol 1996;70:2691–6.
34. Ghany M, Liang TJ. Drug targets and molecular mechanisms of drug resistance in chronic hepatitis B. Gastroenterology 2007;132:1574–85.
35. Bartholomeusz A, Tehan BG, Chalmers DK. Comparisons of the HBV and HIV polymerase, and antiviral resistance mutations. Antivir Ther 2004;9:149–60.
36. Bartenschlager R, Junker-Niepmann M, Schaller H. The P gene product of hepatitis B virus is required as a structural component for genomic RNA encapsidation. J Virol 1990;64:5324–32.
37. Bartenschlager R, Schaller H. Hepadnaviral assembly is initiated by polymerase binding to the encapsidation signal in the viral RNA genome. EMBO J 1992;11: 3413–20.
38. Weber M, Bronsema V, Bartos H, et al. Hepadnavirus P protein utilizes a tyrosine residue in the TP domain to prime reverse transcription. J Virol 1994;68:2994–9.
39. Zoulim F, Seeger C. Reverse transcription in hepatitis B viruses is primed by a tyrosine residue of the polymerase. J Virol 1994;68:6–13.
40. Allen MI, Deslauriers M, Andrews CW, et al. Identification and characterization of mutations in hepatitis B virus resistant to lamivudine. Lamivudine Clinical Investigation Group. Hepatology 1998;27:1670–7.
41. Das K, Xiong X, Yang H, et al. Molecular modeling and biochemical characterization reveal the mechanism of hepatitis B virus polymerase resistance to lamivudine (3TC) and emtricitabine (FTC). J Virol 2001;75:4771–9.
42. Deres K, Schroder CH, Paessens A, et al. Inhibition of hepatitis B virus replication by drug-induced depletion of nucleocapsids. Science 2003;299:893–6.
43. Bourne CR, Finn MG, Zlotnick A. Global structural changes in hepatitis B virus capsids induced by the assembly effector HAP1. J Virol 2006;80:11055–61.
44. Stray SJ, Bourne CR, Punna S, et al. A heteroaryldihydropyrimidine activates and can misdirect hepatitis B virus capsid assembly. Proc Natl Acad Sci U S A 2005; 102:8138–43.
45. Stray SJ, Zlotnick A. BAY 41-4109 has multiple effects on Hepatitis B virus capsid assembly. J Mol Recognit 2006;19:542–8.
46. King RW, Ladner SK, Miller TJ, et al. Inhibition of human hepatitis B virus replication by AT-61, a phenylpropenamide derivative, alone and in combination with (-)beta-L-2',3'-dideoxy-3'-thiacytidine. Antimicrob Agents Chemother 1998;42:3179–86.
47. Delaney WE 4th, Edwards R, Colledge D, et al. Phenylpropenamide derivatives AT-61 and AT-130 inhibit replication of wild-type and lamivudine-resistant strains of hepatitis B virus in vitro. Antimicrob Agents Chemother 2002;46:3057–60.

48. Feld JJ, Colledge D, Sozzi V, et al. The phenylpropenamide derivative AT-130 blocks HBV replication at the level of viral RNA packaging. Antiviral Res 2007; 76:168–77.

49. Block TM, Lu X, Mehta AS, et al. Treatment of chronic hepadnavirus infection in a woodchuck animal model with an inhibitor of protein folding and trafficking. Nat Med 1998;4:610–4.

50. Mehta A, Carrouee S, Conyers B, et al. Inhibition of hepatitis B virus DNA replication by imino sugars without the inhibition of the DNA polymerase: therapeutic implications. Hepatology 2001;33:1488–95.

51. Petersen J, Dandri M, Mier W, et al. Prevention of hepatitis B virus infection in vivo by entry inhibitors derived from the large envelope protein. Nat Biotechnol 2008; 26:335–41.

52. Wilson R, Purcell D, Netter HJ, et al. Does RNA interference provide new hope for control of chronic hepatitis B infection? Antivir Ther 2009;14:879–89.

Hepatitis B Immunology for Clinicians

Kyong-Mi Chang, MD*

KEYWORDS

- Hepatitis B • Innate immunity • Adaptive immunity
- Regulatory T cells • Costimulation • Pathogenesis
- Programmed death 1

GENERAL INTRODUCTION TO INNATE AND ADAPTIVE IMMUNE RESPONSE

The balance between the virus and the host defense mechanisms defines the course of viral infection and disease pathogenesis. To survive, the virus must enter the host, reach its target organ, enter the appropriate cellular compartment, establish replication within the cell, and spread to other cells while avoiding host immune recognition. For the host, various immune mechanisms exist to prevent, limit, and/or eliminate viral infection and spread, preferably without undue collateral damage to itself. Persistent viruses such as hepatitis B virus (HBV) have successful immune evasion mechanisms whereby the host immune defense is selectively circumvented in favor of viral survival. Furthermore, the host-virus interactions may evolve further over chronic infection with additional host, environmental, and viral factors, thus defining the long-term disease outcome.

Pathogen entry into the host (eg, beyond the epithelial barrier) can activate the complement cascade and tissue phagocytes within a few hours. This can be followed by the early induced but nonadaptive responses that are triggered through innate pattern recognition receptors (eg, toll-like receptors [TLRs]) that recognize pathogen-associated molecular patterns (PAMPs) shared by groups of related microbes. This response can involve the neutrophils, macrophages, natural killer (NK) cells, natural killer T (NKT) cells, dendritic cells (DC), and soluble factors including interferons (IFN) and various cytokines and chemokines (REF). Collectively, they contribute to the control of initial infection in a nonspecific manner, without a long-term immunologic memory.

This work was supported in part by NIH UO1 DK082866 and NIH RO1 AI047519
Division of Gastroenterology, Philadelphia VA Medical Center & University of Pennsylvania School of Medicine, University and Woodland Avenues, Philadelphia, PA 19104, USA
* A412/A424 Medical Research Building, Philadelphia VA Medical Center, Philadelphia, PA 19104.
E-mail address: kmchang@mail.med.upenn.edu

IFNs

IFNs belong to the class II family of alpha-helical cytokines. They can be divided into type I (IFNα/β), type II (IFNγ) and type III (IFNλ). Most cells can make IFNβ in response to viral and bacterial pathogens on pathogen-sensing via the membrane-bound TLRs and cytoplasmic RNA helicases (eg, retinoic acid–induced gene I [RIG-I] and melanoma differentiation-associated gene 5 [MDA5]), which results in downstream activation of IFN-regulatory factor 3 (IRF3) and IRF7 followed by IFNβ transcription. Plasmacytoid dendritic cells (pDC) are the major producers of IFNα (up to 1000-fold compared with other cells), although IFNα production can also be up-regulated in myeloid DC (mDC). Binding of IFNα/β to its cell surface receptor activates the downstream IFN-signaling pathway that ultimately leads to the induction of numerous IFN-stimulated genes (ISGs) that mediate a wide array of biologic activities (eg, antiviral, immune modulatory, antiproliferative, antiangiogenic, and antitumor effects).

Type I IFNs can affect all phases of the viral life cycle including entry/uncoating, transcription, RNA stability, translation, maturation, assembly, and release. Three major known IFNα/β-induced antiviral pathways include the dsRNA-dependent protein kinase R (PKR), the 2′,5′-adenylate synthetase system and the Mx proteins. Type I IFNs can also enhance viral protein synthesis, transcription, and replication while enhancing degradation of viral nucleic acid. In addition, type I IFNs can enhance NK cell activity, up-regulate major histocompatibility complex (MHC) expression (especially class I MHC relevant for CD8 T-cell response), influence T- and B-cell development (including isotype switching for B cells), and modulate DC function.

As for type II and III IFNs, IFNγ is often considered in the context of adaptive immune response as a key antiviral T-cell cytokine (although innate immune cells can also secrete IFNγ). IFNλ may have an important role in viral infection with some overlap with IFNα/β in downstream cellular pathways, although our knowledge is still evolving for this relatively new cytokine. IFNλ expression has been detected in various cell types including DCs, macrophages, and cancer cell lines as well as the virus-infected liver. However, its target effect may be more restricted based on its receptor expression but it seems to have some overlap with the IFNα/β pathways.[1]

NK Cells

NK cells are large granular lymphocytes with antiviral and antitumor activities mediated by direct cell lysis and production of proinflammatory cytokines including IFNγ, tumor necrosis factor alpha (TNFα) and granulocyte macrophage colony-stimulating factor (GM-CSF).[2–4] NK cells can be identified by their expression pattern of CD56 (a neural cell adhesion molecule) and CD16 (an Fc receptor). NK cell function is defined by inhibitory and activating receptors that interact with class I HLA molecules on target cells. NK inhibitory receptors include the C-lectin type receptor CD94/NKG2A, LIR1/ILT2 receptors, and killer cell immunoglobulinlike receptors (KIRs). NK-activating receptors include CD16 FcgRIII, NKG2D, the natural cytotoxicity receptors (NCRs) NKp44, NKp46, and NKp30, and truncated alleles of KIRs lacking intracellular immunoreceptor tyrosine-based inhibitory motifs. The coordinated interactions of inhibitory and activating receptors on NK cells with their target cell ligands determine the activation state, viability, and killing potential of NK cells. Cross-talk between NK cells and other immune subsets (eg, DC and T cells) can further influence the adaptive immune response.[5–8]

NKT Cells

NKT cells are innate lymphocytes that express markers of NK cells and T cells (eg, CD56, CD3). NKT cells recognize glycolipid antigens presented by CD1 molecules and can lyse target cells by the perforin and Fas/Fas-ligand pathway. They also secrete proinflammatory (eg, IFNγ) and regulatory (eg, IL-4) cytokines. NKT cells are enriched in the liver with a regulatory effect during hepatic inflammation.

DCs

DCs bridge innate and adaptive immune responses and the major antigen-presenting cells (APC) that prime the adaptive immune response. Circulating DCs include myeloid DCs (mDC) and plasmacytoid DCs (pDC). MDCs express CD11c and produce IL-12 that can enhance the Th1 response and NK cytotoxicity. pDCs express IL3 receptor (CD123) and produce large amounts of type I IFN that can mediate direct antiviral effects and activate NK cytotoxicity.[9] DC dysfunction can result in reduced antigen-specific T-cell response and antiviral cytokine production with potential pathogenetic relevance (as in human immunodeficiency virus [HIV]).[10–12]

Kupffer Cells

Kupffer cells (KCs) are liver-specific macrophages. They can contribute to immune activity within the liver, potentially presenting antigens and producing proinflammatory cytokines. KCs can also modulate NK cell activation in a TLR-dependent manner to enhance immune tolerance and activation within the liver.[13]

Adaptive Immune Response

The adaptive immune response is specific to the antigenic sequence encoded by the infecting pathogen (epitopes), unlike the innate response, which recognizes common molecular patterns shared by various pathogens. Adaptive immunity is mediated by humoral B-cell and cellular T-cell responses that are activated by APCs including DCs.

B-cell response

B cells mediate the humoral adaptive immunity by producing antibodies. Neutralizing antibodies can limit viral spread and promote resolution of viral infection by directly binding and eliminating the circulating virions or blocking virus entry into target cells. Protection afforded by neutralizing antibody is the basis of successful vaccine strategies and passive immunization using hyperimmune globulins. A subset of IL-10–producing regulatory B cells has also been described, expanding the role of B cells.[14]

T-cell response

The virus-specific CD4 and CD8 T cells may be initially activated (or primed) in the primary lymphoid organs on encountering their target viral sequence presented on the surface of the professional APC as short peptides embedded within the MHC. They can then migrate to the site of infection (eg, the liver) to exert their antiviral activity. CD4 T cells recognize exogenously peptide antigens presented by class II MHC molecules on APC, interacting only with class II cells (eg, immune cells such as DCs, B cells, and macrophages). CD4 T cells provide an important regulatory role by activating DCs to prime CD8 T cells, producing antiviral cytokines and providing T-cell help for B cells. By contrast, CD8 T cells (also called cytotoxic T lymphocytes [CTL]) are the foot soldiers of the cell-mediated immune system, recognizing and directly killing the infected cells (via apoptosis through perforin/granzyme and/or the fas/fasL pathway) that display endogenously synthesized viral antigens presented by the class I MHC molecules. CD8 T cells can also cure virus-infected cells in a noncytolytic manner by secreting potent antiviral cytokines.[15] Unlike CD4 T cells, CD8 T cells can recognize most cells including the hepatocytes because class I MHC is expressed on most cells.

In general, a vigorous T-cell response is associated with viral clearance and disease resolution, whereas a weak response is associated with viral persistence and disease progression. T cells can be classified by their cytokine profile as type 1 (IL-2, IFNγ); type 2 (IL-4, 5, 10 and 13); type 3 (TGFβ); type 0 (IFNγ and IL-4); Tr1 (IL-10) with type I response typically associated with a more favorable outcome in viral infection.

Mechanisms of T-cell tolerance and dysfunction
There has been increasing knowledge about immune regulatory mechanisms for antigen-specific effector T-cell response.

One such mechanism involves inhibitory receptors that are directly expressed on T cells to suppress their efficient activation, including programmed death 1 (PD-1) and CTL-associated antigen 4 (CTLA-4). PD-1 and CTLA-4 are inhibitory receptors within the CD28/B7 family of costimulatory molecules, and they are up-regulated on activated and/or exhausted T cells. Binding of PD-1 to its ligands PD-L1 (B7-H4) and PD-L2 (B7-DC). PD-1/PD-ligand interactions can inhibit T-cell proliferation and cytokine secretion[16,17] and promote immune tolerance.[18,19] Although PD-1 expression is up-regulated on exhausted virus-specific T cells during acute and chronic infection, blockade of the PD-1/PD-ligand interaction can restore their effector function. Similarly, binding of CTLA-4 to its ligands (B7-1, B7-2) can suppress T-cell function, whereas blockade of CTLA-4 signaling can reverse T-cell dysfunction. Combined PD-1 and CTLA-4 blockade can provide further synergistic enhancement of intrahepatic hepatitis C virus (HCV)-specific T-cell function compared with individual PD-1 or CTLA-4 blockade. These findings raise the possibility that immune inhibitory blockade may have potential therapeutic application to enhance immune function during chronic viral infection.

A second mechanism involves the induction of immune regulatory cells (eg, CD25+ Tregs and IL-10+ Tr1 cells) that can suppress effector T-cell function. CD4+CD25+ T cells (also termed CD25+ Tregs) are naturally occurring, thymic-derived T cells that represent 5% to 10% of peripheral CD4 T cells and mediate immune tolerance via direct cell-cell contact. Their role in immune regulation is apparent by organ-specific autoimmune diseases that occur on CD25+ Treg depletion and are reversed by their repletion.[20,21] CD25+ Tregs also regulate immune response to pathogens including chronic HCV, HBV, and HIV infection.[22] Another group of regulatory T cells includes the IL-10–secreting Tr1 cells.[23] They are distinct from the CD25+ Tregs, can include CD4 and CD8 T cells, and mediate T-cell suppression via IL-10. IL-10 is a regulatory cytokine secreted by various cell subsets (eg, monocytes, macrophages, and DCs) to limit the inflammatory responses.[24,25] IL-10 can inhibit IFNα production by activated pDC,[26,27] induce a tolerogenic phenotype in DC that can be reversed by PD-1/PD-ligand blockade,[28] and mediate T-cell suppression during chronic viral infection that can be reversed by IL-10/IL010R blockade.[29,30] Collectively, these immune regulatory pathways may contribute to effector T-cell dysfunction in chronic viral infection and their counter-regulation may be critical to a durable response to HBV therapy.

INNATE AND ADAPTIVE IMMUNE RESPONSES IN HBV INFECTION
Innate Immune Response and HBV

HBV does not induce a type I IFN response during acute infection
Multiple innate pathways (eg, TLR, NK/NKT, APCs) can be activated to suppress HBV replication, as shown in HBV-transgenic mice.[15,31,32] HBV replication can also be

suppressed by IFNα, as apparent in patients infected with HBV who are undergoing antiviral therapy. However, gene expression profiling of chimpanzees acutely infected with HBV showed a remarkable lack of type I IFN response in vivo in association with viremia (**Fig. 1**), in contrast to HCV which showed a characteristic type I IFN response.[33,34] The lack of type I IFN induction during acute HBV infection was also observed in a cohort of patients with acute HBV infection[35] and in primary hepatocyte culture following HBV exposure in vitro.[36] These findings suggest that HBV can fly under the radar without triggering a type I IFN response during acute infection.

HBV does activate other innate immune components (NK, NKT, KC, IL-10) during acute infection

Despite the apparent lack of type I IFN response, HBV infection is resolved in most adults with acute HBV infection. HBV can activate other components of the innate defense system [37] including KCs that secrete IL-6[36] and NK/NKT cells with proinflammatory and antiviral effects.[38] **Fig. 2** shows the dynamic changes in NK and NKT cell activation early in the course of acute HBV infection.[39] Early production of immune regulatory cytokine IL-10 was also observed in patients with acute hepatitis B in association with attenuated NK/NKT cell response, consistent with an antiinflammatory role for IL-10.[35]

The course of chronic HBV infection may be defined by changes in innate immune components

Chronic HBV infection (CHB) is associated with changes in innate immune parameters. Unlike the scenario in acute HBV infection, patients with CHB can have increased serum IFNα levels during hepatitis flares.[40] The underlying mechanism for this difference in type I IFN response between acute and chronic HBV infection is not clear. However, hepatitis flares in patients with CHB coincide with increased serum levels of IL-8 and IFNα that may contribute to liver inflammation and hepatocyte injury by up-regulating NK expression of TNF-related apoptosis-inducing ligand (TRAIL) and hepatocyte expression of TRAIL death-inducing receptor. CHB is also associated with mDC and/or pDC dysfunction that may be reversed by therapeutic virus suppression with potential implications for the adaptive immune response.[41,42] Collectively, multiple innate immune pathways are induced during acute and chronic HBV infection, thus shaping the course of infection.

Adaptive Immune Response and HBV

The onset of adaptive immune response is delayed in acute HBV infection

Adaptive immune response to HBV is detected several weeks after inoculation. Although T-cell activation can be observed during the incubation period (several weeks before clinical symptoms), this contrasts with the onset of the adaptive immune response within several days for vaccinia virus or influenza virus infection. The hepatotropic nature of HBV may play a role here because virus-specific adaptive immune response is also delayed in HCV. Increased mechanisms of immune tolerance may exist within the liver as a result of sampling of numerous gut-derived antigens and microbial products. Nevertheless, the apparent delay in adaptive immune response does not necessarily result in chronicity for HBV because HBV infection is resolved in adults with acute HBV infection, whereas HCV becomes chronic in most adults with acute infection.

Neutralizing HBV envelope-specific antibody (anti-HBs) becomes detectable relatively late in the course of HBV infection as HBsAg titers decrease.[15] This may reflect their binding to circulating virions and HBV envelope proteins (needed for viral elimination), because anti-HBs becomes detectable with the loss of circulating HBsAg.

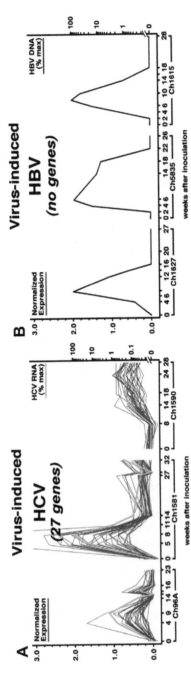

Fig. 1. Liver gene expression profile during acute HBV and acute and chronic HCV infection in chimpanzees. Briefly, gene expression profiles of virus-induced genes from all 3 HCV- or HBV-infected animals were required to positively correlate with viremia with a Pearson's correlation of better than 0.7. HBV liver DNA levels (blue) and HCV serum RNA levels (green) are presented as percentages of the peak level (% max) for the chimpanzee with the highest peak level of HBV and HCV, respectively. (*From* Wieland SF, Chisari FV. Stealth and cunning: hepatitis B and hepatitis C viruses. J Virol 2005;79:9374; with permission.)

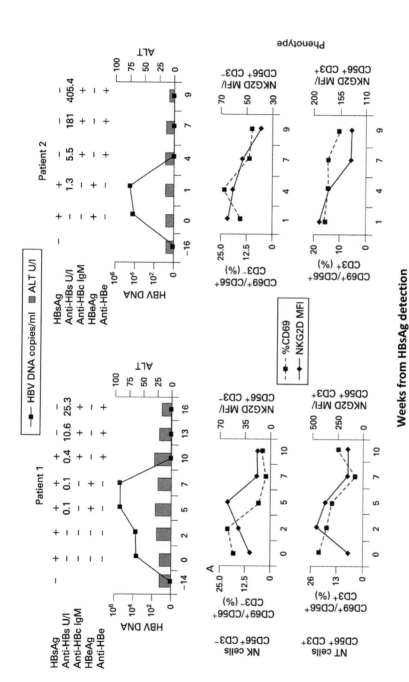

Fig. 2. Phenotypic and functional characterization of NK and CD56+ natural T (NT) cell-mediated responses during acute hepatitis B. *(From* Fisicaro P, Valdatta C, Boni C, et al. Early kinetics of innate and adaptive immune responses during hepatitis B virus infection. Gut 2009;58:976; with permission.)

Neutralizing antibody response to HBV envelope (HBsAg) is the cornerstone of protective humoral immunity following natural infection or vaccination, whereas hepatitis B immunoglobulin provides postexposure prophylaxis and prevents graft infection in liver transplant recipients infected with HBV.

HBV-specific CD4 and CD8 T cells can be readily detected in peripheral blood[43–45] and in the liver[46] of patients during acute HBV infection, displaying activated phenotype and transient functional impairment. With viral clearance and disease resolution, circulating HBV-specific CD8 T cells reduce in frequency as they regain their functional capacity and mature into efficient memory T cells that maintain a broad specificity.[47,48] The antiviral effect of HBV-specific CD8 T cells (cytopathic and perhaps more important noncytolytic effects mediated by antiviral cytokines IFNγ and TNFα) were directly demonstrated in adoptive transfer experiments using transgenic mice that replicate HBV in the liver.[15] A key role for CD8 T cells in HBV clearance and disease pathogenesis was shown in experiments on chimpanzees in which depletion of CD8 (but not CD4) T cells altered the virologic and clinical course,[34] although nonspecific inflammatory cells may also contribute to liver injury.[49]

CONSIDERATIONS IN HBV IMMUNE PATHOGENESIS
What Mediates the Liver Damage in HBV Infection? Is the Virus Directly Cytopathic or is it the Host Immune Response?

Persistent viruses are generally noncytopathic because their continued survival requires a viable host (ie, it does not burn down its own house). HBV replication in experimental infection in chimpanzees (and HBV-replicating transgenic mice) is unaccompanied by any biochemical or histologic evidence for liver injury until host immune responses are activated. Moreover, immunosuppression (eg, by steroids) results in a high level of HBV replication without evidence of liver injury. One exception to this rule may be fibrosing cholestatic hepatitis B in immunosuppressed patients in whom marked hepatocyte injury and ductular reactions are detected without a significant inflammatory component but displaying extremely high levels of HBV replication and the so-called ground glass hepatocytes with massive viral antigen expression.[50] The potential for a cytopathic effect by HBV gene product was also observed in HBV-transgenic mice that overexpressed and retained the large HBV envelope antigen within the endoplasmic reticulum with toxic consequences.[51]

As shown in Fig. 3A, a pathogenetic role for CD8 T cells in liver cell injury was demonstrated by adoptive transfer of virus-specific CD8 T cells that resulted in hepatocyte apoptosis and hepatitis,[15] and by reduced liver inflammation during acute experimental HBV infection in a CD8-depleted chimpanzee.[34] Perforin and Fas death pathways need to be activated simultaneously for CTL-mediated liver injury. CTL-induced liver damage is further amplified by chemokines, neutrophils (with MMPs), and platelets that mediate recruitment of other immune cells (eg, NK, NKT, T/B cells, macrophages, monocytes, DCs) into the liver.[52]

Although CTLs (and the recruited inflammatory cells) contribute to liver cell injury, these interactions also result in the elaboration of antiviral cytokines (eg, IFNγ) that can cure virus-infected hepatocytes, ultimately leading to resolution of HBV infection without fulminant liver failure. **Fig. 3**B shows a schematic of CTL-mediated recognition in which a small number of HBV-infected hepatocytes are killed with concurrent production of potent antiviral T-cell cytokines that can cure HBV infection in a noncytopathic manner from a greater number of hepatocytes. These cytokines can also induce chemokines that promote recruitment of antigen-nonspecific inflammatory cells including neutrophils that elaborate MMPs that further amplify this process.

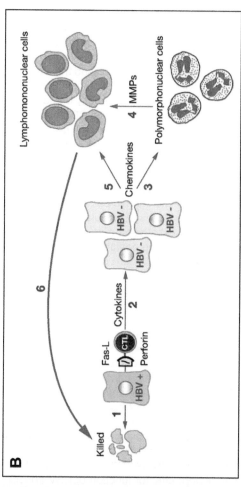

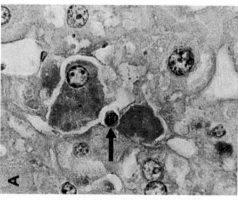

Fig. 3. (A) Bromodeoxyuridine-labeled HBsAg-specific CTL (*arrow*) is identified in association with apoptotic hepatocytes at 4 hours after their adoptive transfer into HBsAg transgenic mice. (*B*) A schema showing CTL-mediated lysis of HBV-infected hepatocytes (1) and release of antiviral cytokines (2) that can cure HBV-infected hepatocytes in a noncytopathic manner while recruiting further nonspecific inflammatory cells via chemokines (5) and neutrophils (6) that induce matrix metalloproteinase (4) to further amplify the inflammatory response (6). (*From* Guidotti LG, Chisari FV. Immunobiology and pathogenesis of viral hepatitis. Annu Rev Pathol 2006;1:31, 33; with permission.)

Immune Mechanisms of HBV Persistence

The precise mechanism of HBV persistence is not fully defined. Although HBV fails to efficiently induce type I IFN response during acute infection, other innate immune response elements (eg, NK and KC) are activated and HBV infection is ultimately resolved in most infected adults. A potential relevance of T cells in the virologic outcome of HBV infection is suggested by the robust antiviral T-cell response detected in patients in whom HBV infection is resolved and the weak or dysfunctional antiviral T-cell response in patients with chronic infection.[53,54] The critical role for CD8 T cells in HBV clearance and liver injury was more directly demonstrated by the prolonged viremia and attenuated liver inflammation in CD8-depleted chimpanzees experimentally infected with HBV.[34] Although therapeutic HBsAg vaccination during lamivudine therapy can enhance antibody and CD4 T-cell responses to HBV envelope, this does not translate to a sustained therapeutic response,[55] further supporting the role of CD8 T cells in HBV clearance. However, it remains unclear how CD8 T cells fail in HBV persistence.

In neonates, HBV infection may become chronic because of an immature immune system, a tolerizing effect of HBV antigens (particularly the soluble HBeAg that crosses the placenta),[56,57] and T-cell exhaustion and/or clonal deletion.[58] Detailed immunologic analysis of HBV infection in the pediatric population is extremely challenging because their small size prohibits large volume blood draw for sufficient lymphocyte isolation. Thus, studies of immune tolerance mechanisms in newborns may need to rely on animal models. Nevertheless, it seems that newborns can mount an effective response to HBV vaccination that can effectively prevent HBV infection with chronic evolution.

In adults, prolonged T-cell activation caused by high levels of viral antigens may result in T-cell exhaustion and anergy or even clonal deletion. The extent of these immune inhibitory pathways may define the course of chronic HBV infection from immune tolerance to immune active and healthy carrier state as well as hepatitis flares. For example, HBV-specific CD8 T cells from patients with chronic HBV infection may be at risk for increased attrition as a result of increased expression of the proapoptotic molecule, Bcl-interacting mediator. During acute hepatitis B, HBV-specific CD8 T cells also display increased PD-1 expression and impaired function that may be reversed with viral clearance.[59] In patients with chronic HBV infection, HBV-specific CD8 T cells are also highly PD-1+ and functionally impaired[60,61] in peripheral blood and the liver. PD-1/PD-ligand blockade can restore effector function of HBV-specific CD8 T cells. HBV persistence has been associated with CTLA-4 in a study of single nucleotide polymorphisms,[62] although its role has not yet been examined functionally in HBV.

HBV persistence has been associated with the induction of CD25+ Tregs that can suppress HBV-specific effector T cells.[63,64] CD25+ Treg frequency was increased in peripheral blood and the liver of patients infected with HBV, and circulating CD25+ Treg frequency correlated with HBV titer.[65] In patients with HBV-associated hepatocellular carcinoma, the circulating Treg frequency also correlated with disease progression and mortality.[66] As for IL-10+ Tr1 response, a global cytokine deviation toward a Th0 phenotype rather than Th1 phenotype has been reported in chronic HBV infection.[67] However, T cells and monocytes from patients infected with HBV can secrete IL-10 in response to HBV core protein[68,69] and a surge in serum IL-10 levels associated with transient inhibition of NK and T-cell response occurs in patients with acute HBV infection.[35]

Viral mutations may contribute to HBV persistence. For example, CD8 T-cell epitope variants that escape CTL recognition and even induce CTL antagonism[70,71] have been identified in patients with CHB.[72] However, ongoing escape mutation was not common in established chronic infection without immune selection pressure.[73] Relevant for therapy, reduced immunogenicity has been associated with antiviral resistance in patients treated with lamivudine,[74] suggesting that HBV drug resistance may have immunologic consequences.

Can HBV Infection be Truly Cleared?

HBV infection can reactivate on significant immunosuppression (eg, steroids and/or transplant immunosuppression) in persons with previous resolution of their infection based on standard serologic assays (eg, −HBsAg, +anti-HBs, normal liver enzymes). It has been shown that minute amounts of HBV DNA can persist for decades after recovery from acute HBV infection, maintaining a level of cell-mediated immune response that may maintain virus control.[75] With increased sensitivity in the HBV DNA quantitation assays, the concept of HBV clearance versus occult infection and persistent infection has been evolving. Thus, the goal in HBV therapy may be control rather than cure of HBV infection.

What is the Role of Cell-mediated Immune Response in the Natural History and Treatment Outcome of Chronic Hepatitis B?

Although HBV-specific CD8 T cells are dysfunctional during chronic HBV infection, an inverse relationship exists between HBV-specific CD8 T-cell response and HBV DNA. For example, HBV-specific CD8 T cells are more easily detected and more functional in HBV carriers with lower viral titer compared with highly viremic patients who display little to no detectable HBV-specific CD8 T-cell response.[43,44] Although HBV-specific T-cell response in CHB infection seems to mostly target the HBV core,[60] HBc-specific CD8 T-cell response (albeit low in frequency) showed a significant inverse association with HBV titer,[72] consistently detectable ex vivo in patients with viral titers less than (but not more than) 10 million copies/mL.

In the liver, HBV-specific CD8 T cells are found in similar numbers in patients displaying immune control (minimal liver inflammation, low HBV DNA) and in patients with active disease (ongoing liver inflammation, high HBV DNA).[76] However, in patients with active disease, HBV-specific CD8 T cells were effectively diluted as a result of massive inflammatory infiltrates to the liver that may be cytopathic without antiviral activity. In this regard, inflammatory cytokines induced during chronic HBV infection can enhance cytopathic activity of NK cells.[40] Thus, ineffective HBV-specific CD8 T cells may contribute to cytopathology by promoting the recruitment of nonspecific inflammatory infiltrate (eg, NK cells) as shown for **Fig. 3**B. It is likely that this is a dynamic process in patients with active chronic hepatitis B or flares.

Conversely, HBV can influence the functionality of HBV-specific T cells. For example, the level of viral antigen has been shown to influence CD8 T-cell function.[77] HBV-specific T-cell function is enhanced when the level of HBV DNA is reduced during antiviral therapy, unlike HCV in which therapeutic IFNα-mediated viral clearance is not routinely associated with virus-specific T-cell augmentation.[78,79] For example, complete virologic response following IFNα therapy was associated with a vigorous and multispecific cytolytic CD8 T-cell response to HBV similar to those in patients with natural HBV clearance.[54] Furthermore, HBV-specific T-cell effector function is enhanced by lamivudine-mediated HBV suppression,[80,81] although this effect is lost with time as viremia recurs with the emergence of lamivudine-resistant mutations.[74] HBV suppression during lamivudine therapy was also associated with increased nonspecific CD4 proliferative T-cell responses, suggesting a more global immune effect associated with HBV suppression.[80–82] A better understanding of the immune modulatory pathways in chronic HBV infection may help in identifying prognostic markers for therapeutic outcome in the long-term.

Active HBV viremia results in the induction of various immune regulatory mechanisms that may be reversed on therapeutic virus suppression, thereby leading to enhanced antiviral effector T-cell response. Prolonged therapeutic HBV suppression may ultimately tip the balance toward sustained HBV control by dampening the immune regulatory pathways and enhancing the immune effector responses. These results suggest that virus-specific T-cell precursors may not be deleted but functionally tolerized in CHB and that therapeutic viral clearance might restore their function.

SUMMARY

HBV infection triggers several innate and adaptive immune responses. Because HBV is largely noncytopathic, host immune response is believed to define the course of HBV infection. HBV does not trigger the type I IFN response during acute infection, but can induce other innate immune subsets (eg, NK, DC). As for adaptive immunity, CD8 T cells play a critical role in HBV clearance, whereas they are functionally suppressed during chronic HB infection via multiple immune regulatory mechanisms (PD-1, CTLA-4, FxP3+ Tregs). Further studies are needed to define the dynamic balance between HBV, the liver, and the innate/adaptive immune response.

REFERENCES

1. Sommereyns C, Paul S, Staeheli P, et al. IFN-lambda (IFN-lambda) is expressed in a tissue-dependent fashion and primarily acts on epithelial cells in vivo. PLoS Pathog 2008;4:e1000017.
2. Carayannopoulos LN, Yokoyama WM. Recognition of infected cells by natural killer cells. Curr Opin Immunol 2004;16:26–33.
3. Kirwan SE, Burshtyn DN. Regulation of natural killer cell activity. Curr Opin Immunol 2007;19:46–54.
4. Long EO, Burshtyn DN, Clark WP, et al. Killer cell inhibitory receptors: diversity, specificity, and function. Immunol Rev 1997;155:135–44.
5. Piccioli D, Sbrana S, Melandri E, et al. Contact-dependent stimulation and inhibition of dendritic cells by natural killer cells. J Exp Med 2002;195:335–41.
6. Gerosa F, Gobbi A, Zorzi P, et al. The reciprocal interaction of NK cells with plasmacytoid or myeloid dendritic cells profoundly affects innate resistance functions. J Immunol 2005;174:727–34.
7. Gerosa F, Baldani-Guerra B, Nisii C, et al. Reciprocal activating interaction between natural killer cells and dendritic cells. J Exp Med 2002;195:327–33.
8. Moretta A. The dialogue between human natural killer cells and dendritic cells. Curr Opin Immunol 2005;17:306–11.
9. Pacanowski J, Kahi S, Baillet M, et al. Reduced blood CD123+ (lymphoid) and CD11c+ (myeloid) dendritic cell numbers in primary HIV-1 infection. Blood 2001;98:3016–21.
10. Boasso A, Shearer GM. Chronic innate immune activation as a cause of HIV-1 immunopathogenesis. Clin Immunol 2008;126:235–42.
11. Desai S, Chaparro A, Liu H, et al. Impaired CCR7 expression on plasmacytoid dendritic cells of HIV-infected children and adolescents with immunologic and virologic failure. J Acquir Immune Defic Syndr 2007;45:501–7.
12. Chehimi J, Campbell DE, Azzoni L, et al. Persistent decreases in blood plasmacytoid dendritic cell number and function despite effective highly active

antiretroviral therapy and increased blood myeloid dendritic cells in HIV-infected individuals. J Immunol 2002;168:4796–801.

13. Tu Z, Bozorgzadeh A, Pierce RH, et al. TLR-dependent cross talk between human Kupffer cells and NK cells. J Exp Med 2008;205:233–44.

14. Bouaziz JD, Yanaba K, Tedder TF. Regulatory B cells as inhibitors of immune responses and inflammation. Immunol Rev 2008;224:201–14.

15. Guidotti LG, Chisari FV. Immunobiology and pathogenesis of viral hepatitis. Annu Rev Pathol Mech Dis 2006;1:23–61.

16. Freeman GJ, Long AJ, Iwai Y, et al. Engagement of the PD-1 immunoinhibitory receptor by a novel B7 family member leads to negative regulation of lymphocyte activation. J Exp Med 2000;192:1027–34.

17. Latchman Y, Wood CR, Chernova T, et al. PD-L2 is a second ligand for PD-1 and inhibits T cell activation. Nat Immunol 2001;2:261–8.

18. Riley JL, June CH. The road to recovery: translating PD-1 biology into clinical benefit. Trends Immunol 2006;28(2):48–50.

19. Freeman GJ, Wherry EJ, Ahmed R, et al. Reinvigorating exhausted HIV-specific T cells via PD-1-PD-1 ligand blockade. J Exp Med 2006;203:2223–7.

20. Shevach EM. CD4+ CD25+ suppressor T cells: more questions than answers. Nat Rev Immunol 2002;2:389–400.

21. Sakaguchi S. Naturally arising CD4+ regulatory t cells for immunologic self-tolerance and negative control of immune responses. Annu Rev Immunol 2004; 22:531–62.

22. Rouse BT, Suvas S. Regulatory cells and infectious agents: detentes cordiale and contraire. J Immunol 2004;173:2211–5.

23. Roncarolo MG, Gregori S, Battaglia M, et al. Interleukin-10-secreting type 1 regulatory T cells in rodents and humans. Immunol Rev 2006;212:28–50.

24. Moore KW, de Waal Malefyt R, Coffman RL, et al. Interleukin-10 and the interleukin-10 receptor. Annu Rev Immunol 2001;19:683–765.

25. Vicari AP, Trinchieri G. Interleukin-10 in viral diseases and cancer: exiting the labyrinth? Immunol Rev 2004;202:223–36.

26. Zou W, Borvak J, Wei S, et al. Reciprocal regulation of plasmacytoid dendritic cells and monocytes during viral infection. Eur J Immunol 2001;31:3833–9.

27. McKenna K, Beignon AS, Bhardwaj N. Plasmacytoid dendritic cells: linking innate and adaptive immunity. J Virol 2005;79:17–27.

28. Brown JA, Dorfman DM, Ma FR, et al. Blockade of programmed death-1 ligands on dendritic cells enhances T cell activation and cytokine production. J Immunol 2003;170:1257–66.

29. Brooks DG, Trifilo MJ, Edelmann KH, et al. Interleukin-10 determines viral clearance or persistence in vivo. Nat Med 2006;12:1301–9.

30. Ejrnaes M, Filippi CM, Martinic MM, et al. Resolution of a chronic viral infection after interleukin-10 receptor blockade. J Exp Med 2006;203:2461–72.

31. Kakimi K, Guidotti LG, Koezuka Y, et al. Natural killer T cell activation inhibits hepatitis B virus replication in vivo. J Exp Med 2000;192:921–30.

32. Kimura K, Kakimi K, Wieland S, et al. Activated intrahepatic antigen-presenting cells inhibit hepatitis B virus replication in the liver of transgenic mice. J Immunol 2002;169:5188–95.

33. Wieland S, Thimme R, Purcell RH, et al. Genomic analysis of the host response to hepatitis B virus infection. Proc Natl Acad Sci U S A 2004;101:6669–74.

34. Thimme R, Wieland S, Steiger C, et al. CD8(+) T cells mediate viral clearance and disease pathogenesis during acute hepatitis B virus infection. J Virol 2003;77: 68–76.

35. Dunn C, Peppa D, Khanna P, et al. Temporal analysis of early immune responses in patients with acute hepatitis B virus infection. Gastroenterology 2009;137: 1289–300.

36. Hosel M, Quasdorff M, Wiegmann K, et al. Not interferon, but interleukin-6 controls early gene expression in hepatitis B virus infection. Hepatology 2009; 50:1773–82.

37. Durantel D, Zoulim F. Innate response to hepatitis B virus infection: observations challenging the concept of a stealth virus. Hepatology 2009;50: 1692–5.

38. Guy CS, Mulrooney-Cousins PM, Churchill ND, et al. Intrahepatic expression of genes affiliated with innate and adaptive immune responses immediately after invasion and during acute infection with woodchuck hepadnavirus. J Virol 2008;82:8579–91.

39. Fisicaro P, Valdatta C, Boni C, et al. Early kinetics of innate and adaptive immune responses during hepatitis B virus infection. Gut 2009;58:974–82.

40. Dunn C, Brunetto M, Reynolds G, et al. Cytokines induced during chronic hepatitis B virus infection promote a pathway for NK cell-mediated liver damage. J Exp Med 2007;204:667–80.

41. van der Molen RG, Sprengers D, Biesta PJ, et al. Favorable effect of adefovir on the number and functionality of myeloid dendritic cells of patients with chronic HBV. Hepatology 2006;44:907–14.

42. Zhang Z, Zhang H, Chen D, et al. Response to interferon-alpha treatment correlates with recovery of blood plasmacytoid dendritic cells in children with chronic hepatitis B. J Hepatol 2007;47:751–9.

43. Maini MK, Boni C, Lee CK, et al. The role of virus-specific CD8(+) cells in liver damage and viral control during persistent hepatitis B virus infection. J Exp Med 2000;191:1269–80.

44. Maini MK, Boni C, Ogg GS, et al. Direct ex vivo analysis of hepatitis B virus-specific CD8(+) T cells associated with the control of infection. Gastroenterology 1999;117:1386–96.

45. Penna A, Artini M, Cavalli A, et al. Long-lasting memory T cell responses following self-limited acute hepatitis B. J Clin Invest 1996;98:1185–94.

46. Sprengers D, van der Molen RG, Kusters JG, et al. Analysis of intrahepatic HBV-specific cytotoxic T-cells during and after acute HBV infection in humans. J Hepatol 2006;45:182–9.

47. Penna A, Chisari FV, Bertoletti A, et al. Cytotoxic T lymphocytes recognize an HLA-A2-restricted epitope within the hepatitis B virus nucleocapsid antigen. J Exp Med 1991;174:1565–70.

48. Rehermann B, Fowler P, Sidney J, et al. The cytotoxic T lymphocyte response to multiple hepatitis B virus polymerase epitopes during and after acute viral hepatitis. J Exp Med 1995;181:1047–58.

49. Sitia G, Isogawa M, Iannacone M, et al. MMPs are required for recruitment of antigen-nonspecific mononuclear cells into the liver by CTLs. J Clin Invest 2004;113:1158–67.

50. Thung SN. Histologic findings in recurrent HBV. Liver Transpl 2006;12:S50–3.

51. Chisari FV. Hepatitis B virus transgenic mice: insights into the virus and the disease. Hepatology 1995;22:1316–25.

52. Iannacone M, Sitia G, Isogawa M, et al. Platelets mediate cytotoxic T lymphocyte-induced liver damage. Nat Med 2005;11:1167–9.

53. Rehermann B. Immune responses in hepatitis B virus infection. Semin Liver Dis 2003;23:21–38.

54. Rehermann B, Lau D, Hoofnagle JH, et al. Cytotoxic T lymphocyte responsiveness after resolution of chronic hepatitis B virus infection. J Clin Invest 1996;97: 1655–65.

55. Vandepapeliere P, Lau GK, Leroux-Roels G, et al. Therapeutic vaccination of chronic hepatitis B patients with virus suppression by antiviral therapy: a randomized, controlled study of co-administration of HBsAg/AS02 candidate vaccine and lamivudine. Vaccine 2007;25:8585–97.

56. Chen MT, Billaud JN, Sallberg M, et al. A function of the hepatitis B virus precore protein is to regulate the immune response to the core antigen. Proc Natl Acad Sci U S A 2004;101:14913–8.

57. Chen M, Sallberg M, Hughes J, et al. Immune tolerance split between hepatitis B virus precore and core proteins. J Virol 2005;79:3016–27.

58. Wherry EJ, Ahmed R. Memory CD8 T-cell differentiation during viral infection. J Virol 2004;78:5535–45.

59. Boettler T, Panther E, Bengsch B, et al. Expression of the interleukin-7 receptor alpha chain (CD127) on virus-specific CD8+ T cells identifies functionally and phenotypically defined memory T cells during acute resolving hepatitis B virus infection. J Virol 2006;80:3532–40.

60. Boni C, Fisicaro P, Valdatta C, et al. Characterization of hepatitis B virus (HBV)-specific T-cell dysfunction in chronic HBV infection. J Virol 2007;81:4215–25.

61. Fisicaro P, Valdatta C, Massari M, et al. Antiviral intrahepatic T-cell responses can be restored by blocking programmed death-1 pathway in chronic hepatitis B. Gastroenterology 2009;138(2):682–93.

62. Thio CL, Mosbruger TL, Kaslow RA, et al. Cytotoxic T-lymphocyte antigen 4 gene and recovery from hepatitis B virus infection. J Virol 2004;78:11258–62.

63. Stoop JN, van der Molen RG, Baan CC, et al. Regulatory T cells contribute to the impaired immune response in patients with chronic hepatitis B virus infection. Hepatology 2005;41:771–8.

64. Franzese O, Kennedy PT, Gehring AJ, et al. Modulation of the CD8+-T-cell response by CD4+ CD25+ regulatory T cells in patients with hepatitis B virus infection. J Virol 2005;79:3322–8.

65. Xu D, Fu J, Jin L, et al. Circulating and liver resident CD4+CD25+ regulatory T cells actively influence the antiviral immune response and disease progression in patients with hepatitis B. J Immunol 2006;177:739–47.

66. Fu J, Xu D, Liu Z, et al. Increased regulatory T cells correlate with CD8 T-cell impairment and poor survival in hepatocellular carcinoma patients. Gastroenterology 2007;132:2328–39.

67. Bertoletti A, D'Elios MM, Boni C, et al. Different cytokine profiles of intrahepatic T cells in chronic hepatitis B and hepatitis C virus infections. Gastroenterology 1997;112:193–9.

68. Hyodo N, Tajimi M, Ugajin T, et al. Frequencies of interferon-gamma and interleukin-10 secreting cells in peripheral blood mononuclear cells and liver infiltrating lymphocytes in chronic hepatitis B virus infection. Hepatol Res 2003;27: 109–16.

69. Hyodo N, Nakamura I, Imawari M. Hepatitis B core antigen stimulates interleukin-10 secretion by both T cells and monocytes from peripheral blood of patients with chronic hepatitis B virus infection. Clin Exp Immunol 2004;135:462–6.

70. Bertoletti A, Costanzo A, Chisari FV, et al. Cytotoxic T lymphocyte response to a wild type hepatitis B virus epitope in patients chronically infected by variant viruses carrying substitutions within the epitope. J Exp Med 1994; 180:933–43.

71. Bertoletti A, Sette A, Chisari FV, et al. Natural variants of cytotoxic epitopes are T-cell receptor antagonists for antiviral cytotoxic T cells. Nature 1994;369:407–10.
72. Webster GJ, Reignat S, Brown D, et al. Longitudinal analysis of CD8+ T cells specific for structural and nonstructural hepatitis B virus proteins in patients with chronic hepatitis B: implications for immunotherapy. J Virol 2004;78:5707–19.
73. Rehermann B, Pasquinelli C, Mosier SM, et al. Hepatitis B virus (HBV) sequence variation of cytotoxic T lymphocyte epitopes is not common in patients with chronic HBV infection. J Clin Invest 1995;96:1527–34.
74. Mizukoshi E, Sidney J, Livingston B, et al. Cellular immune responses to the hepatitis B virus polymerase. J Immunol 2004;173:5863–71.
75. Rehermann B, Ferrari C, Pasquinelli C, et al. The hepatitis B virus persists for decades after patients' recovery from acute viral hepatitis despite active maintenance of a cytotoxic T-lymphocyte response. Nat Med 1996;2:1104–8.
76. Bertoletti A, Maini M, Williams R. Role of hepatitis B virus specific cytotoxic T cells in liver damage and viral control. Antiviral Res 2003;60:61–6.
77. Gehring AJ, Sun D, Kennedy PT, et al. The level of viral antigen presented by hepatocytes influences CD8 T-cell function. J Virol 2007;81:2940–9.
78. Kaplan DE, Sugimoto K, Ikeda F, et al. T-cell response relative to genotype and ethnicity during antiviral therapy for chronic hepatitis C. Hepatology 2005;41:1365–75.
79. Rahman F, Heller T, Sobao Y, et al. Effects of antiviral therapy on the cellular immune response in acute hepatitis C. Hepatology 2004;40:87–97.
80. Boni C, Penna A, Ogg GS, et al. Lamivudine treatment can overcome cytotoxic T-cell hyporesponsiveness in chronic hepatitis B: new perspectives for immune therapy. Hepatology 2001;33:963–71.
81. Boni C, Penna A, Bertoletti A, et al. Transient restoration of anti-viral T cell responses induced by lamivudine therapy in chronic hepatitis B. J Hepatol 2003;39:595–605.
82. Boni C, Bertoletti A, Penna A, et al. Lamivudine treatment can restore T cell responsiveness in chronic hepatitis B. J Clin Invest 1998;102:968–75.

Antiviral Therapy for Chronic Hepatitis B

Syed-Mohammed R. Jafri, MD, Anna Suk-Fong Lok, MD*

KEYWORDS

- Interferon • Nucleos(t)ide analogs • Hepatitis B virus DNA
- Hepatitis B e antigen • Cirrhosis

The goal of antiviral therapy for chronic hepatitis B is to prevent the development of cirrhosis, liver failure, and hepatocellular carcinoma (HCC). Not all patients with chronic hepatitis B virus (HBV) infection will develop these outcomes, and for those who do, outcomes may not occur until after several decades of infection. Therefore, more easily measurable end points, including viral suppression, hepatitis B e antigen (HBeAg) loss, hepatitis B surface antigen (HBsAg) loss, alanine aminotransferase (ALT) normalization, and improvement in liver histology, are used to determine the success of treatment.[1,2] Studies of patients who had not undergone treatment found that persistently active HBV replication or hepatic inflammation, as reflected by high serum HBV DNA, elevated ALT, or the presence of HBeAg, are associated with increased risk of progressive liver disease.[3–7] Therefore, indications for chronic hepatitis B treatment are based on HBV replication status and activity and stage of liver disease.[1,8–10]

During the past decade, the number of approved hepatitis B treatments increased from one parenteral therapy, conventional interferon, to seven medications, including five orally administered nucleos(t)ide analogs and two interferon preparations: conventional and pegylated interferons. The availability of medications that have potent antiviral activity and are safe for use in patients with cirrhosis and liver failure has broadened the indications for hepatitis B treatment. This expansion in turn led to a recent decline in the number of patients with HBV added to the liver transplant waiting list[11] and a decrease in age-adjusted rates of HBV-related deaths in the United States.[12] Despite these advances, many questions regarding hepatitis B treatment remain: (1) when to start treatment, (2) which medication to begin with, and (3) when treatment can be stopped. This article focuses on initial treatment, whereas management of patients with antiviral resistance will be covered in the article by Locarnini elsewhere in this issue.

Financial Disclosures: Syed-Mohammed Jafri has no financial disclosures or funding support. Anna Suk-Fong Lok has received research grants from Schering, Roche, Bristol-Myers Squibb, GlaxoSmithKline, and Gilead and has served on advisory panels for Bristol-Myers Squibb, Roche, and Gilead.
Division of Gastroenterology, University of Michigan Health System, 3912 Taubman Center, SPC 5362, Ann Arbor, MI 48109, USA
* Corresponding author.
E-mail address: aslok@umich.edu

WHEN TO START TREATMENT

The decision to start antiviral therapy in patients with life-threatening HBV–liver disease, who have little to lose and much to gain, is easy. The decision is more difficult in patients with mild or early-stage liver disease, because current HBV treatment does not eradicate the virus and most patients will require many years of treatment, and some lifelong, to prevent clinical outcomes. **Box 1** summarizes the indications for HBV treatment.

Life-Threatening Liver Disease

In patients with life-threatening liver disease, such as acute liver failure, decompensated cirrhosis, or severe exacerbation of chronic hepatitis B, the decision to start treatment is obvious. Although randomized controlled trials of antiviral therapy in these settings are lacking, the benefits of oral antiviral therapy have been shown in cohort studies and case series.[13,14] These studies showed that antiviral therapy can stabilize liver function, allowing patients to proceed to liver transplant, and in some instances liver function improved to the extent that patients could be taken off the transplant waiting list. For patients who undergo liver transplantation, decrease in serum HBV DNA levels before transplantation also decreases the risk of HBV recurrence after transplant.

Patients with life-threatening liver disease should undergo antiviral therapy regardless of serum HBV DNA and ALT levels, and treatment should be initiated as soon as possible because clinical benefit may take 3 to 6 months.[14]

Compensated Cirrhosis

Patients with compensated cirrhosis are at risk of developing hepatic decompensation and HCC. A landmark double-blind, randomized, placebo-controlled trial of lamivudine in patients with bridging fibrosis or cirrhosis and high levels of HBV replication (HBe-positive and/or serum HBV DNA >700,000 genome equivalents/mL [roughly 140,000 IU/mL]) showed that lamivudine treatment significantly reduced the risk of disease progression, defined as an increase in Child-Turcotte-Pugh score by 2 or

---

Box 1
Indications for hepatitis B virus therapy

Clearly indicated

Acute liver failure

Cirrhosis and clinical complications

Advanced fibrosis with high serum HBV DNA

HBsAg-positive status with chemotherapy or immunosuppressive therapy planned

Might be indicated

HBeAg-positive or -negative chronic hepatitis B with active liver disease

Not routinely indicated

HBeAg-positive in immune tolerance phase

HBeAg-negative in inactive carrier phase

Data from Sorrell MF, Belongia EA, Costa J, et al. National Institutes of Health Consensus Development Conference Statement: management of hepatitis B. Ann Intern Med 2009;150(2):104–10.

more points, onset of clinical decompensation, or development of HCC.[15] A significant difference in primary end point between the treatment and control groups (7.8% vs 17.7%; $P = .001$) was observed after a mean of 32.6 months, prompting an independent data safety and monitoring board to recommend termination of the trial. This trial also found a significant difference in the incidence of HCC between the groups (3.9% vs 7.4%; $P = .047$).

These data have led many experts to recommend antiviral treatment for all patients with compensated cirrhosis; however, the benefits of antiviral therapy on clinical outcomes in patients with compensated cirrhosis and low serum HBV DNA have not been proven. The American Association for the Study of Liver Diseases (AASLD) guidelines recommended that patients with compensated cirrhosis and serum HBV DNA greater than 2000 IU/mL undergo antiviral therapy.[8] A lower cutoff in serum HBV DNA was selected because recent data showed that persistently high serum HBV DNA is associated with increased risk of liver-related mortality and HCC, and the risk increases when serum HBV DNA exceeds 10,000 copies/mL (~2000 IU/mL).[5,6]

Liver Disease Without Advanced Fibrosis

A unique aspect of chronic HBV infection is the fluctuations in HBV replication and activity of liver disease, reflecting changes in balance between the virus and the host immune response. The course of chronic HBV infection is generally divided into four phases, although not all patients experience all phases, and the duration each patient remains in each phase is highly variable.[16] Among patients who do not have advanced fibrosis, antiviral treatment is recommended for those in the immune clearance or reactivation phase but not for those in the immune tolerance or inactive carrier phase. The decision to start treatment is based on HBV replication status and activity or stage of liver disease, and is modulated by the age of the patient, HBeAg status, and other factors, such as patient preference (**Figs. 1** and **2**).[17]

Immune tolerance phase

The immune tolerance phase is characterized by the presence of HBeAg, normal ALT, and high HBV DNA levels. Antiviral therapy is not recommended for patients in this

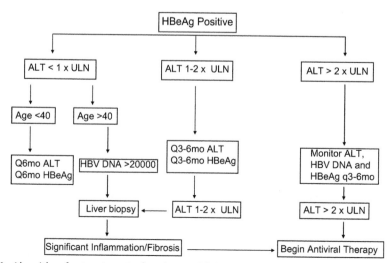

Fig. 1. Algorithm for treatment of patients with HBeAg-positive hepatitis B.

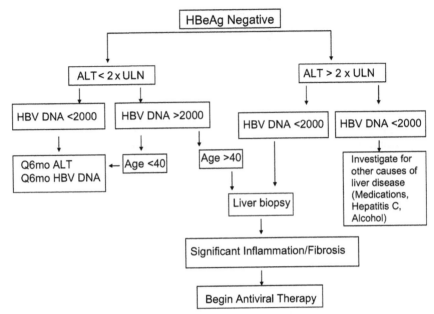

Fig. 2. Algorithm for treatment of patients with HBeAg-negative hepatitis B.

phase because most have minimal inflammation and little or no fibrosis.[18,19] In addition, follow-up studies showed that fibrosis progression and clinical outcomes were infrequent in patients who remained in this phase.[18,20] Another reason for deferring treatment is that antiviral treatment is less efficacious during this phase. Numerous studies have shown that treatment (interferon and nucleos(t)ide analog)-induced HBeAg seroconversion is uncommon (<10% after 1 year of treatment) in patients with normal or minimally elevated (1–2 times upper limit of normal [ULN]) ALT.[21] A recent study found that a lower percentage of patients with HBeAg-positive hepatitis with minimally elevated ALT experienced virologic (undetectable serum HBV DNA) or biochemical (ALT normalization) responses during entecavir treatment compared with those with ALT greater than two times ULN.[22] Therefore, treatment guidelines recommend that patients in the immune tolerance phase be monitored.

Several studies found that persistently high serum HBV DNA level is associated with an increased risk of cirrhosis, liver failure, and HCC.[5,6,23] However, most patients in those studies were HBeAg-negative and more than half were older than 40 years at enrollment. A long-term follow-up study of 508 patients with HBeAg-positive hepatitis found that delayed HBeAg clearance (after age 40 years) is associated with an increased risk of cirrhosis and HCC.[7] These data have prompted treatment guidelines to recommend liver biopsies and consideration of antiviral therapy for patients who remain in the immune tolerance phase after the age of 40 years.

Immune clearance phase or typical HBeAg-positive hepatitis
The immune clearance phase is characterized by the presence of HBeAg, high/fluctuating serum HBV DNA levels, persistent or intermittent elevation of ALT, and evidence of necroinflammation on liver biopsies. Some patients undergo spontaneous HBeAg seroconversion and enter the inactive carrier phase after a short immune clearance phase. Other patients may experience recurrent hepatitis flares and may progress

to cirrhosis or hepatic decompensation while they are still in the immune clearance phase. Therefore, treatment guidelines recommend that patients in the immune clearance phase be monitored for 3 to 6 months to determine if they will undergo spontaneous HBeAg seroconversion.[8,9] Patients who remain HBeAg-positive with ALT greater than two times ULN after 3 to 6 months should undergo antiviral treatment. Treatment should be commenced immediately in patients with icteric flares or evidence of hepatic decompensation.

Inactive carrier phase

The inactive carrier phase is characterized by the absence of HBeAg, persistently normal ALT, and low or undetectable serum HBV DNA. Patients in the inactive carrier phase have a favorable prognosis, particularly if they enter this phase at a young age and before irreversible liver damage occurs.[24] Recent studies showed that patients with high normal ALT (0.5–1 times ULN) have an increased risk of liver mortality compared with those with low normal ALT (<0.5 times ULN).[25] Several studies also showed that significant liver disease can be found in patients with persistently normal ALT.[26,27] However, many of these studies were based on one or two ALT values, and most of the histologic studies were conducted in patients with serum HBV DNA greater than 4 to 5 $\log_{10}$ copies/mL. No evidence supports the hypothesis that antiviral therapy will alter the outcome of patients who are truly in the inactive carrier phase.

Reactivation phase or HBeAg-negative chronic hepatitis

The reactivation phase is characterized by the absence of HBeAg, intermittent or persistently elevated ALT, and HBV DNA levels that vary from undetectable to as high as 8 to 9 $\log_{10}$ IU/mL. Most patients have precore or core promoter variants that prevent or decrease the production of HBeAg. Patients in this phase often have a fluctuating course. Therefore, serial monitoring is needed to determine if a patient is in the inactive carrier or reactivation phase. Treatment is recommended once patients are deemed to have HBeAg-negative chronic hepatitis because many have advanced liver disease, and sustained spontaneous remission is rare.

Other Factors to Consider

Other factors may influence the timing of treatment initiation. Age (a surrogate for the duration of infection) is an important consideration, particularly in patients with HBeAg-positive hepatitis who have normal or minimally elevated ALT levels. An important consideration for young female patients is the immediacy of their plans to become pregnant. Although two of the approved nucleos(t)ide analogs are listed as class B drugs (telbivudine and tenofovir), data on the safety of antiviral therapy during the first trimester of pregnancy are limited. The Antiretroviral Pregnancy Registry has been tracking spontaneously reported maternal and fetal outcomes in women receiving oral nucleosides since 1989. As of July 2009, 10,803 pregnancies had been reported in which the mother had received an oral nucleoside analog for HBV or HIV infection.[28] The prevalence of birth defects in babies who had been exposed to lamivudine in the first trimester was 2.9% (96 of 3314) and was 2.4% (18 of 756) in those exposed to tenofovir. These findings were similar to those of population controls. However, only outcomes of live births were recorded. The frequency of spontaneous abortions and the impact of exposure to nucleos(t)ides on growth and development of the babies have not been studied.

Data regarding the risk of birth defects associated with entecavir, adefovir, or telbivudine are limited because of the small number of live births reported. Antiviral treatment should be recommended for women who present with life-threatening liver disease and those with compensated cirrhosis and high levels of HBV DNA. For patients who do not have advanced fibrosis, the decision regarding when to start antiviral therapy should balance the immediacy of pregnancy plans, the anticipated duration of treatment, and the likelihood of spontaneous improvement. For example, patients with HBeAg-positive hepatitis with minimally elevated ALT may defer treatment because the short-term prognosis is favorable and many years of treatment will be required to achieve HBeAg seroconversion. All patients should be monitored so that treatment can be initiated if their liver disease becomes more active.

Familial clustering of HCC has been reported in several studies. Whether genetic, viral, or environmental factors contribute to familial clustering of HCC, and how the risk of HCC can be assessed in patients with a family history are unknown. Although putting patients with chronic HBV infection and a family history of HCC on antiviral therapy may seen reasonable, no data support that antiviral therapy in patients who otherwise do not meet criteria for treatment will derive any clinical benefit.

Patients with chronic HBV infection who undergo immunosuppressive therapy or chemotherapy for other medical conditions are at risk for exacerbating hepatitis secondary to reactivation of HBV replication.[29] Prophylactic antiviral therapy is recommended for all patients with HBsAg-positive hepatitis who require long-term immunosuppressive therapy. Reactivation of HBV replication may also occur in patients with HBsAg-negative, hepatitis B core antibody (anti-HBc)–positive hepatitis, but the risk is substantially lower.[30] Although data are limited, most experts would recommend prophylactic antiviral therapy for patients with HBsAg-negative, anti-HBc–positive hepatitis undergoing high-risk treatments such as chemotherapy for hematologic malignancies or bone marrow transplantation; rituximab for any reason; or long-term steroids.

WHAT SHOULD BE THE INITIAL THERAPY?

Once a decision is made to initiate treatment, the next question is which medication to use. The decision regarding nucleos(t)ide versus interferon therapy is based on patient characteristics and preference. **Table 1** summarizes the pros and cons of interferon and nucleos(t)ide analog therapy. Interferon therapy is not recommended for patients with hepatic decompensation, immunosuppression, or medical or psychiatric contraindications. The main advantage of interferon is that it is administered for a finite duration. Interferon also seems to be associated with a higher rate of HBsAg loss, although this benefit is mainly seen in patients with genotype A infection. Some studies found that interferon-induced HBeAg seroconversion is more durable than nucleoside-induced HBeAg seroconversion, but a direct comparison has not been performed. The main disadvantages of interferon are the need for parenteral administration and

Table 1
Comparison of interferon alfa and nucleos(t)ide analog therapy

Treatment	Interferon-Alfa	Nucleos(t)ide Analog
Route	Subcutaneous injection	Oral
Duration of treatment	Finite (12 mo)	Years to lifelong
Antiviral activity	Moderate	Strong, varies by therapy
HBsAg loss	1%–3% after 1 y	0%–1% after 1 y, varies by therapy
Antiviral resistance	None	0%–25% after 1 y
Adverse effects	Frequent	Rare

the frequent side effects. Nucleos(t)ide analogs are administered orally and are very well tolerated, but viral relapse is common when treatment is withdrawn, necessitating long durations of treatment with associated risks of antiviral drug resistance.

Nucleos(t)ide Analog Therapy

The nucleos(t)ide analogs approved for use in hepatitis B fall into three groups: L-nucleosides, including lamivudine and telbivudine; acyclic nucleoside phosphonates, including tenofovir and adefovir; and deoxyguanosine analogs, including entecavir. Mutations associated with drugs in one group confer at least some resistance to other drugs within the same group and, in some instances, also reduce the sensitivity to drugs in other groups. The selection of the initial treatment should be based on antiviral activity and risk of antiviral resistance. **Table 2** compares the rates of response and resistance to the five approved nucleos(t)ide analogs. Entecavir, telbivudine, and tenofovir have more potent antiviral activity, followed by lamivudine and then adefovir. Entecavir and tenofovir have higher genetic barrier to resistance (ie, lower rate of resistance) followed by adefovir, telbivudine, and then lamivudine.

All five approved nucleos(t)ide analogs are well tolerated; however, like other nucleoside analogs, the potential exists for mitochondrial toxicity and lactic acidosis. The need for vigilance is underscored by the recent withdrawal of clevudine, which was reported to be associated with mitochondrial toxicity and myopathy during long-term use.[31,32] Adefovir and tenofovir were reported to be associated with nephrotoxicity in up to 3% of patients after 3 to 5 years of continuous treatment,[33,34] and with renal tubular dysfunction, including Fanconi syndrome. Telbivudine has been reported to be associated with myalgia/myositis and peripheral neuropathy in 1.4% and 0.28% of patients after 3 years of treatment, respectively. The risk of peripheral neuropathy was markedly increased in patients who underwent combination therapy of telbivudine and peginterferon (18.75%).[35,36] A recent case series found that entecavir was associated with a high rate of lactic acidosis when used in patients with severe liver decompensation.[37]

Nucleos(t)ide analogs are most appropriate for patients with decompensated liver disease, those with contraindications to interferon, and those who are willing to commit to long durations of treatment. Among the five approved medications, entecavir and tenofovir have the best profile regarding efficacy, safety, and drug resistance. Entecavir is preferred in patients with other medical conditions that are associated with increased risks of renal insufficiency, whereas tenofovir is preferred in young female patients who might be contemplating pregnancy and patients who might have been exposed to lamivudine in the past. Lamivudine and telbivudine should not be used as first-line therapy because of high rates of drug resistance, whereas adefovir is largely superseded by tenofovir because of its weak antiviral activity.

Interferon

Interferon is contraindicated in patients with decompensated cirrhosis because of the risks of severe sepsis and worsening of liver failure.[38,39] It is also not advisable in patients with severe exacerbations of chronic hepatitis B or acute liver failure, and in those undergoing immunosuppressive or cancer chemotherapy. Interferon may be used in patients with compensated cirrhosis who have normal synthetic function and no evidence of portal hypertension. In the large registration trials of pegylated interferon alfa-2a, ALT flares (>5 times ULN) occurred, but none resulted in hepatic decompensation despite the fact that 18% of HBeAg-positive and 31% of patients with HBeAg-negative hepatitis treated with pegylated interferon monotherapy had advanced fibrosis or compensated cirrhosis.[40,41]

Table 2
Response rates to approved therapies for HBeAg-positive and -negative chronic hepatitis B[a]

	Lamivudine	Adefovir	Entecavir	Telbivudine	Tenofovir	Pegylated Interferon[a]	Pegylated Interferon and Lamivudine[a]	Placebo
HBeAg-positive								
At week 48 or 52								
Histology improved	49–62	53–68	72	65	74	38	41	25
Undetectable HBV DNA	40–44	21	67	60	76	25	69	0–16
HBeAg seroconversion	16–21	12	21	22	21	27	24	4–6
HBsAg loss	<1	0	2	0	3	3	3	0
During extended treatment (y)[b]								
Undetectable HBV DNA	NA	39 (5)	94 (5)	79 (4)	72 (3)	13[c] (4.5)	26[c] (4.5)	NA
HBeAg seroconversion	47 (3)	48 (5)	41 (5)	42 (4)	26 (3)	37%[c] (4.5)	36[c] (4.5)	NA
HBsAg loss	0–3 (2–3)	2 (5)	5 (2)	1 (2)	8 (3)	8[c] (4.5)	15[c] (4.5)	NA
HBeAg-negative								
At week 48 or 52								
Histology Improved	60–66	64–69	70	67	72	48	38	33
Undetectable HBV DNA	60–73	51	90	88	93	63	87	0

Histologic improvement defined as a ≥2-point decrease in necroinflammatory score and no worsening of fibrosis score.
Abbreviation: NA, not available.
[a] Liver biopsy performed 24 weeks after stopping treatment.
[b] Time-point in which response was assessed in years.
[c] Assessment performed off treatment.
Data from Lok AS, McMahon BJ. Chronic hepatitis B. Update 2009. AASLD Practice Guidelines. Available at: http://www.aasld.org. Accessed November 25, 2009.

Several studies have examined the predictors of response to pegylated interferon therapy to refine the selection of patients for interferon treatment. In a retrospective analysis of 721 patients from pooled data of two phase III trials of pegylated interferon in patients with HBeAg-positive hepatitis, high ALT, low HBV DNA, female sex, older age, and absence of previous interferon therapy were predictors of response. The best outcomes occurred in patients with genotype A with high ALT or low HBV DNA and those with genotypes B or C with both high ALT and low HBV DNA.[42]

Interferon differs from nucleos(t)ide analogs in that it has immunomodulatory and antiviral effects, which may account for the higher rate of HBsAg loss and durable viral suppression.[42,43] Three years after treatment, 28% of patients with HBeAg-negative hepatitis treated with pegylated interferon had HBV DNA levels of 10,000 copies/mL or less versus 15% of patients treated with lamivudine ($P = .039$), and 8.7% of pegylated interferon–treated patients cleared HBsAg compared with none treated with lamivudine alone.[43]

These data indicate that the best candidates for interferon therapy are young patients who have no medical or psychiatric comorbidities and who do not wish to commit to a long duration of treatment. For patients with HBeAg-positive hepatitis, genotyping should be considered, and those who have genotype A infection should be encouraged to try interferon.[42]

De Novo Combination Therapy

De novo combination therapy has been advocated because of the potential for additive or synergistic antiviral activity and prevention of antiviral drug resistance. Most clinical trials on de novo combination therapy have used lamivudine as the nucleos(t)ide analog. These studies showed that neither combination of lamivudine and pegylated interferon or lamivudine and another nucleos(t)ide analog had a clear advantage over monotherapy regarding speed or extent of viral suppression. The main advantage of these combination therapies was a reduction in the rate of lamivudine resistance. Given the low rate of antiviral drug resistance associated with entecavir or tenofovir monotherapy, the benefit of de novo combination therapy will be limited.

Combination of pegylated interferon and nucleos(t)ide analog therapy

Compared with pegylated interferon alone, the addition of lamivudine to pegylated interferon resulted in more marked viral suppression during treatment, but this difference was not maintained when treatment was stopped.[40,41,44] De novo combination of pegylated interferon and lamivudine was also associated with a lower rate of lamivudine resistance compared with lamivudine monotherapy, but lamivudine resistance was not encountered in patients who underwent pegylated interferon monotherapy. A clinical trial of combination therapy with pegylated interferon and telbivudine was terminated because of a high rate of peripheral neuropathy. Clinical trials are ongoing of combination therapy with pegylated interferon and entecavir, with simultaneous versus staggered onset of the two medications and varying duration of entecavir.

Combination of nucleos(t)ide therapies

Currently, all of the approved oral drugs for hepatitis B target the HBV polymerase. Furthermore, mutations associated with resistance to one drug may confer resistance to another. To date, clinical trials of de novo combination of nucleos(t)ide analogs have shown no additive or synergistic antiviral activity, and that resistance to lamivudine is reduced but not completely prevented. Until drugs with new targets are available, the role of de novo combination of oral antiviral agents is limited.

A phase II trial comparing combination of telbivudine and lamivudine versus telbivudine alone and lamivudine alone found that combination therapy was similar or inferior to telbivudine alone.[45] This result is likely related to the fact that both lamivudine and telbivudine are L-nucleosides, and mutations to one drug have cross-resistance to the other drug.

Another trial compared combination of lamivudine and adefovir with lamivudine alone in 115 patients with HBeAg-positive hepatitis.[46] Initial decline in serum HBV DNA levels was not different between the groups. At week 104, the percent of patients with undetectable serum HBV DNA and HBeAg seroconversion were also comparable. Patients who underwent combination therapy had a significantly lower rate of lamivudine resistance (15%) than the group that received only lamivudine therapy (43%). The high rate of lamivudine resistance in the de novo combination therapy group was surprising and is likely related to the weak antiviral activity of adefovir.

MONITORING PATIENTS UNDERGOING THERAPY

Monitoring patients during treatment allows response, tolerability, and adherence to be assessed. All patients should be closely monitored during treatment and for at least 24 weeks after treatment withdrawal, because hepatitis flares associated with viral relapse may occur, necessitating immediate resumption of treatment. Long-term monitoring is important to detect late relapses, the durability of response, and the rate of HBsAg loss. HCC surveillance should be performed according to guideline recommendations even in patients who have maintained viral suppression on treatment or sustained virologic response off treatment.

Patients receiving pegylated interferon should be assessed clinically at 12- to 24-week intervals. Tests for blood counts and hepatic panel should be performed every 4 weeks initially and then every 4 to 12 weeks. Serum HBV DNA should be tested every 12 weeks. Thyroid hormone should be checked every 12 weeks during treatment and for 24 weeks after stopping treatment. HBeAg and HBe antibody (anti-HBe) should be tested every 12 to 24 weeks in patients who were HBeAg-positive initially. HBsAg should be tested every 24 to 48 weeks. Retrospective analysis of patients treated with pegylated interferon found that decline in HBsAg titer during the first 12 or 24 weeks is predictive of long-term viral suppression and HBsAg loss.[47] Similarly, decline in HBeAg titer was predictive of HBeAg loss in patients who were HBeAg-negative before treatment.[48] These data suggest that monitoring of HBeAg or HBsAg titer may help in tailoring the duration of treatment and identifying those who are unlikely to benefit from continued interferon treatment; however, these findings must be verified in prospective studies before they can be applied clinically.

Patients undergoing nucleos(t)ide analog therapy should be assessed clinically every 24 weeks and the importance of adherence to medications emphasized. Serum HBV DNA and ALT should be monitored at 12 and 24 weeks, and every 12 to 24 weeks thereafter. Patients with suboptimal viral response may benefit from the addition of a second drug. This "road-map" approach was derived from experience using lamivudine and telbivudine, which have high rates of antiviral drug resistance. The applicability of this strategy and the definition of *suboptimal response* in patients receiving entecavir or tenofovir have not been determined. HBeAg and anti-HBe should be tested every 24 to 48 weeks in patients who were HBeAg-positive before treatment, and HBsAg should be tested annually in those who are HBeAg negative. Patients receiving adefovir or tenofovir should also be tested for serum creatinine at least every 24 weeks, and more often in older patients and those with medical comorbidities that are associated with increased risk of renal insufficiency.

WHEN CAN TREATMENT BE STOPPED?

Ideally, antiviral therapy should be continued until HBsAg loss is confirmed; however, the likelihood that this will occur is low, with rates of approximately 3% to 5% after 3 to 5 years of nucleos(t)ide analog therapy and roughly 5% to 10% at 5 years after completing a course of pegylated interferon therapy.

Pegylated Interferon

Pegylated interferon is administered for a finite duration because the immunomodulatory effects of interferon may persist after treatment is stopped. Based on results of phase III clinical trials, the recommended duration of treatment is 48 weeks for patients with HBeAg-positive and -negative hepatitis. Ongoing studies will determine whether a shorter duration of treatment will suffice for patients with HBeAg-positive hepatitis with favorable characteristics, eg, genotype A infection, high ALT and low HBV DNA. Recent studies suggest that monitoring of HBsAg titer may identify a subset of patients who experience a slow response who may benefit from a longer duration of treatment, and patients who do not experience response in whom continued treatment is futile. The validity of a tailored approach similar to what is currently used in patients with hepatitis C must be confirmed in prospective studies.

Nucleos(t)ide Analogs

Nucleos(t)ide analogs are administered until the desired end point is achieved. For patients who had decompensated cirrhosis, lifelong treatment is recommended because of concerns for fatal flares when treatment is withdrawn. For patients who had compensated cirrhosis, some experts also recommend lifelong treatment. In view of data showing reversal of fibrosis and cirrhosis in patients who have maintained viral suppression after 3 to 5 years of antiviral therapy, it would be reasonable to recommend cessation of treatment in patients who are documented to have reversal of cirrhosis and those who have confirmed HBsAg loss, provided that these patients are closely monitored so that treatment can be promptly reinstituted if a biochemical or clinical relapse occurs.

For patients HBeAg-positive hepatitis who have not experienced progression to cirrhosis, the AASLD guidelines recommended that treatment should be continued until the patient has achieved HBeAg seroconversion (HBeAg-negative, anti-HBe–positive, and undetectable serum HBV DNA) and completed at least 6 months of additional therapy.[8] Many experts have questioned the validity of HBeAg seroconversion as a treatment end point, citing that some patients remain viremic after HBeAg seroconversion, and that reversion to HBeAg positivity occurs in up to 50% of patients when treatment is stopped. These arguments indicate that many patients will enter the inactive carrier phase and remain in that phase for months, years, or decades after HBeAg seroconversion. Therefore, discontinuing treatment in patients who completed consolidation therapy after achieving HBeAg seroconversion is reasonable as long as these patients continue to be monitored.

For patients with HBeAg-negative hepatitis who have not experienced progression to cirrhosis, the therapeutic end point is unclear. Relapse is common even in those who completed 2 years treatment and had undetectable serum HBV DNA for at least 1 year.[49] Preliminary data from one small study found that among 33 patients who discontinued treatment after 4 to 5 years of adefovir therapy and had undetectable serum HBV DNA for at least 3 years, 18 had sustained clinical remission and 9 lost HBsAg during a mean of 5 years of posttreatment follow-up.[50] However, all of the patients experienced viral relapse shortly after treatment was stopped, but serum HBV DNA levels decreased to low or undetectable levels during off-treatment follow-up. Additional studies are needed to confirm these data and to determine predictors of sustained clinical remission. This information may help in selecting when treatment can be stopped, thus sparing some patients from lifelong treatment.

REFERENCES

1. Sorrell MF, Belongia EA, Costa J, et al. National institutes of health consensus development conference statement: management of hepatitis B. Ann Intern Med 2009;150(2):104–10.
2. Lok AS, McMahon BJ. Chronic Hepatitis B. Update 2009. AASLD Practice Guidelines. Available at: http://www.aasld.org. Accessed November 25, 2009.
3. Liaw YF, Tai DI, Chu CM, et al. The development of cirrhosis in patients with chronic type B hepatitis: a prospective study. Hepatology 1988;8:493–6.
4. Fattovich G, Brollo L, Giustina G, et al. Natural history and prognostic factors for chronic hepatitis type B. Gut 1991;32:284–8.
5. Iloeje UH, Yang H, Jen CL, et al. Risk and predictors of mortality associated with chronic hepatitis B infection. Clin Gastroenterol Hepatol 2007;5(8):921–31.
6. Chen CJ, Yang HI, Su J, et al. Risk of hepatocellular carcinoma across a biological gradient of serum hepatitis B virus DNA level. JAMA 2006;295:65–73.
7. Chen YC, Chu CM, Liaw YF. Age-specific prognosis following spontaneous hepatitis B e antigen seroconversion in chronic hepatitis B. Hepatology 2010;51(2):435–44.
8. Lok AS, McMahon BJ. Chronic hepatitis B. Hepatology 2007;45:507–39.
9. European Association for the Study of the Liver. EASL Clinical practice guidelines: management of chronic hepatitis B. J Hepatol 2009;50(2):227–42.
10. Liaw YF, Leung N, Kao JH, et al. Asian-Pacific consensus statement on the management of chronic hepatitis B: a 2008 update. Hepatol Int 2008;2:263–83.
11. Kim WR, Terrault NA, Pedersen RA, et al. Trends in waiting list registration for liver transplantation for viral hepatitis in the United States. Gastroenterology 2009;137(5):1680–6.
12. Ruhl CE, Everhart JE. Elevated serum alanine aminotransferase and gamma-glutamyltransferase and mortality in the United States population. Gastroenterology 2009;136(2):477–85.
13. Yao FY, Terrault NA, Freise C, et al. Lamivudine treatment is beneficial in patients with severely decompensated cirrhosis and actively replicating hepatitis B infection awaiting liver transplantation: a comparative study using a matched, untreated cohort. Hepatology 2001;34:411–6.
14. Fontana RJ, Hann HW, Perrillo RP, et al. Determinants of early mortality in patients with decompensated chronic hepatitis B treated with antiviral therapy. Gastroenterology 2002;123:719–27.
15. Liaw YF, Sung JJ, Chow WC, et al. Lamivudine for patients with chronic hepatitis B and advanced liver disease. N Engl J Med 2004;351:1521–31.
16. Yim HJ, Lok AS. Natural history of chronic hepatitis B virus infection: what we knew in 1981 and what we know in 2005. Hepatology 2006;43(2 Suppl 1):S173–81.
17. Degertekin B, Lok AS. Indications for therapy in hepatitis B. Hepatology 2009;49(S5):S129–37.
18. Hui CK, Leung N, Yuen ST, et al. Natural history and disease progression in Chinese chronic hepatitis B patients in immune-tolerant phase. Hepatology 2007;46(2):395–401.

19. Andreani T, Serfaty L, Mohand D, et al. Chronic hepatitis B virus carriers in the immunotolerant phase of infection: histologic findings and outcome. Clin Gastroenterol Hepatol 2007;5(5):636–41.

20. Chu CM, Hung SJ, Lin J, et al. Natural history of hepatitis B e antigen to antibody seroconversion in patients with normal serum aminotransferase levels. Am J Med 2004;116:829–34.

21. Perrillo RP, Lai CL, Liaw YF, et al. Predictors of HBeAg loss after lamivudine treatment for chronic hepatitis B. Hepatology 2002;36(1):186–94.

22. Wu IC, Lai CI, Han SH, et al. Efficacy of entecavir in chronic hepatitis B patients with mildly elevated ALT and biopsy-proven histologic damage. Hepatology 2010;51(4):1185–9.

23. Iloeje UH, Yang HI, Su J, et al. Predicting liver cirrhosis risk based on the level of circulating hepatitis B viral load. Gastroenterology 2006;130:678–86.

24. Manno M, Cammà C, Schepis F, et al. Natural history of chronic HBV carriers in northern Italy: morbidity and mortality after 30 years. Gastroenterology 2004; 127(3):756–63.

25. Yuen MF, Yuan HJ, Wong DK, et al. Prognostic determinants for chronic hepatitis B in Asians: therapeutic implications. Gut 2005;54(11):1610–4.

26. Lai M, Hyatt BJ, Nasser I, et al. The clinical significance of persistently normal ALT in chronic hepatitis B infection. J Hepatol 2007;47(6):760–7.

27. Kumar M, Sarin SK, Hissar S, et al. Virologic and histologic features of chronic hepatitis B virus-infected asymptomatic patients with persistently normal ALT. Gastroenterology 2008;134(5):1376–84.

28. The Antiretroviral Pregnancy Registry. Available at: http://www.apregistry.com. Accessed December 10, 2009.

29. Hoofnagle JH. Reactivation of hepatitis B. Hepatology 2009;49(Suppl 5): S156–65.

30. Lok AS, Liang RH, Chiu EK, et al. Reactivation of hepatitis B virus replication in patients receiving cytotoxic therapy: report of a prospective study. Gastroenterology 1991;100:182–8.

31. Seok JI, Lee DK, Lee CH, et al. Long-term therapy with clevudine for chronic hepatitis B can be associated with myopathy characterized by depletion of mitochondrial DNA. Hepatology 2009;49(6):2080–6.

32. Kim BK, Oh J, Kwon SY, et al. Clevudine myopathy in patients with chronic hepatitis B. J Hepatol 2009;51(4):829–34.

33. Marcellin P, Chang TT, Lim SG, et al. Long-term efficacy and safety of adefovir dipivoxil for the treatment of hepatitis B e antigen-positive chronic hepatitis B. Hepatology 2008;48(3):750–8.

34. Hadziyannis SJ, Tassopoulos NC, Heathcote EJ, et al. Long-term therapy with adefovir dipivoxil for HBeAg-negative chronic hepatitis B for up to 5 years. Gastroenterology 2006;131(6):1743–51.

35. Avila C, Laeufle R, Bao W. CK elevation during chronic hepatitis B (CHB) treatment with telbivudine: experience from the combined globe (NV-02B-007/ CLDT600A2302) and NV-02B-015(015) study clinical safety database. Presented at the 19th Asian Pacific Association for the Study of the Liver (APASL). Hong Kong, February 13–16, 2009.

36. Goncalves J, Laeufle R, Avila C. Increased risk with combination of telbivudine and pegylated-interferon Alfa-2A in study CLDT600A2406, compared to uncommon rate with telbivudine monotherapy from the Novartis global database. J Hepatol 2009;50:S329.

37. Lange CM, Bojunga J, Hofmann WP, et al. Severe lactic acidosis during treatment of chronic hepatitis B with entecavir in patients with impaired liver function. Hepatology 2009;50(6):2001–6.

38. Hoofnagle JH, Di Bisceglie AM, Waggoner JG, et al. Interferon alfa for patients with clinically apparent cirrhosis due to chronic hepatitis B. Gastroenterology 1993;104:1116–21.

39. Perrillo R, Tamburro C, Regenstein F, et al. Low-dose, titratable interferon alfa in decompensated liver disease caused by chronic infection with hepatitis B virus. Gastroenterology 1995;109:908–16.

40. Lau GK, Piratvisuth T, Luo KX, et al. Peginterferon alfa-2A, lamivudine, and the combination for HBeAg-positive chronic hepatitis B. N Engl J Med 2005;352: 2682–95.

41. Marcellin P, Lau GK, Bonino F, et al. Peginterferon alfa-2a alone, lamivudine alone, and the two in combination in patients with HBeAg-negative chronic hepatitis B. N Engl J Med 2004;351:1206–17.

42. Buster EH, Hansen BE, Lau GK, et al. Factors that predict response of patients with hepatitis B e antigen-positive chronic hepatitis B to peginterferon-alfa. Gastroenterology 2009;137(6):2002–9.

43. Marcellin P, Bonino F, Lau GK, et al. Sustained response of hepatitis B e antigen-negative patients 3 years after treatment with peginterferon alfa-2a. Gastroenterology 2009;136(7):2388.

44. Janssen HL, van Zonneveld M, Senturk H, et al. Pegylated interferon alfa-2b alone or in combination with lamivudine for HBeAg-positive chronic hepatitis B: a randomised trial. Lancet 2005;365:123–9.

45. Lai CL, Leung N, Teo EK, et al. A 1-year trial of telbivudine, lamivudine, and the combination in patients with hepatitis B e antigen-positive chronic hepatitis B. Gastroenterology 2005;129(2):528–36.

46. Sung JJ, Lai JY, Zeuzem S, et al. Lamivudine compared with lamivudine and adefovir dipivoxil for the treatment of HBeAg-positive chronic hepatitis B. J Hepatol 2008;48(5):728–35.

47. Moucari R, Mackiewicz V, Lada O, et al. Early serum HBsAg drop: A strong predictor of sustained virological response to pegylated interferon alfa-2a in HBeAg-negative patients. Hepatology 2009;49(4):1151–7.

48. Brunetto MR, Moriconi F, Bonino F, et al. Hepatitis B virus surface antigen levels: a guide to sustained response to peginterferon alfa-2a in HBeAg-negative chronic hepatitis B. Hepatology 2009;49(4):1141–50.

49. Fung SK, Wong F, Hussain M, et al. Sustained response after a 2-year course of lamivudine treatment of hepatitis B e antigen-negative chronic hepatitis B. J Viral Hepat 2004;11(5):432–8.

50. Hadziyannis S, Sevastianos V, Rapti I. Outcome of HBeAg-negative chronic hepatitis B (CHB) 5 years after discontinuation of long term adefovir dipivoxil (ADV) treatment. J Hepatol 2009;50(S1):S9–10.

Drug Resistance in Antiviral Therapy

Stephen Locarnini, MBBS, PhD, FRC[Path][a,*], Scott Bowden, PhD[b]

KEYWORDS

- Hepatitis B virus • Antiviral resistance • Nucleoside analog
- Nucleotide analog • Multidrug resistance
- Reverse transcriptase

Hepatitis B virus (HBV) is a DNA-containing virus and a prototypical member of the family *Hepadnaviridae*. HBV is distantly related to the retroviruses and replicates its genome by the reverse transcription of an RNA intermediate, the pregenomic RNA. The 3.2-kb partially double-stranded DNA genome is organized into four overlapping but frame-shifted open-reading frames (ORFs; **Fig. 1**). The longest of these encodes the viral reverse transcriptase (rt)-polymerase (P ORF). The second ORF, referred to as the "envelope" or "surface" (S) ORF, encodes the viral surface proteins and is contained within the P ORF. Two smaller ORFs that encode the precore-core proteins and the X protein, respectively, also partially overlap the P ORF. The viral life cycle of HBV is relatively well characterized considering the lack of a robust and readily available permissive infection cell model.[1]

The unique replication strategy of HBV provides it with at least two selective advantages. First, the HBV covalently closed circular (ccc) DNA-minichromosome that acts as the major transcriptional template for the virus is inherently stable. Second, the error-prone HBV rt polymerase causes a high nucleotide substitution rate, generating a population of viral variants or quasispecies capable of rapidly responding to endogenous (host immune response) and exogenous selection (antiviral therapy or during viral transmission) pressures. This reservoir of variants (quasispecies) provides HBV with a survival advantage by already having a pool of pre-existing escape mutants to the immune response (precore or HBeAg-escape); prophylactic vaccines (vaccine escape); and antiviral therapy (drug resistance).

Under normal circumstances HBV infection and subsequent replication within hepatocytes is generally not cytopathic. The clinical course and outcome of persistent HBV replication is determined, however, by the generation and selection of viral escape mutants. Frequent unsuccessful attempts by the host's immune response to clear

[a] Department of R&MD, Victorian Infectious Diseases Reference Laboratory, 10 Wreckyn Street, North Melbourne, Victoria 3051, Australia
[b] Department of Molecular Microbiology, Victorian Infectious Diseases Reference Laboratory, 10 Wreckyn Street, North Melbourne, Victoria 3051, Australia
* Corresponding author.
E-mail address: stephen.locarnini@mh.org.au

Clin Liver Dis 14 (2010) 439–459
doi:10.1016/j.cld.2010.05.004
1089-3261/10/$ – see front matter © 2010 Elsevier Inc. All rights reserved.

liver.theclinics.com

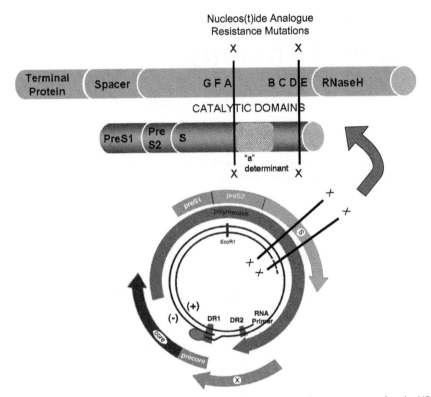

Fig. 1. The implications of a circular genome. Polymerase-envelope gene overlap in HBV highlighting that antiviral drug-resistant changes in the polymerase can cause potentially important changes in HBsAg with all the nucleos(t)ide analogs (NA) currently available. The "a" determinant (the neutralization domain of HBV) is also highlighted.

wild-type and escape mutants of HBV from infected hepatocytes leads to the necroinflammation and liver damage typically associated with chronic hepatitis B (CHB).[2] Furthermore, active HBV replication correlates with active liver disease, and a number of long-term natural history studies from Asia have recently established the direct relationship between HBV replication and clinical outcomes. The serum HBV DNA level is the best available indicator of HBV replication. Elevations of HBV DNA above 10^4 copies/mL have been shown to be a risk predictor for the development of liver cirrhosis and hepatocellular carcinoma in a dose-dependent manner.[2–4]

ANTIVIRAL DRUG RESISTANCE: BACKGROUND

The management of CHB has advanced significantly during the past 10 years because of the development of safe and efficacious oral antiviral nucleos(t)ide analogs (NAs). Approved medications include lamivudine (LMV), a synthetic deoxycytidine analog with an unnatural L-conformation, and the related L-nucleoside, telbivudine (LdT; β-L-thymidine). A second group, the acyclic phosphonates, includes adefovir dipivoxil (ADV), a prodrug for the acyclic 2′-deoxyadenosine monophosphate analog adefovir, and the structurally similar tenofovir (TFV). A third group of agents contains a D-cyclopentane sugar moiety and includes the most potent anti-HBV drug discovered to date, the deoxyguanosine analog entecavir (ETV).[5] This structural classification of the NA is useful clinically because it does help to categorize the patterns and pathways of NA drug resistance (see later).

Antiviral drug resistance is defined as the reduced susceptibility of a virus to the inhibitory effect of a drug, and results from a process of adaptive mutations under the selection pressure of antiviral therapy. Two types of mutations have been identified: primary resistance mutations, which are directly responsible for the associated drug-resistance, and secondary or compensatory mutations. The latter probably occur to facilitate replication competence because primary resistance mutations are usually associated with a reduction in replication fitness for the virus. Compensatory mutations are important because they reduce the deleterious effects to the virus associated with acquisition of primary drug-resistant mutations.[6]

The virologic indications of emergence of drug-resistant virus include the detection of an increasing viral load, typically greater than 1 $\log_{10}$ IU/mL from nadir,[7–9] or the presence of known genotypic markers of drug resistance encoded within the viral polymerase. Other parameters are an increasing serum alanine aminotransferase (ALT) level and clinical deterioration. There are several risk factors associated with the development of NA resistance. These include a high level of HBV DNA, high serum levels of ALT, and high body mass index.[10–12] Prior therapy with NA, and inadequate viral suppression during therapy, has also been shown to predict drug resistance.[11,13–15] Transmission of drug-resistant variants in newly infected patients is also likely to predispose to more rapid resistance once treatment is initiated, as has been shown for HIV infection (see later).

CAUSES OF ANTIVIRAL DRUG RESISTANCE

The development of antiviral drug resistance depends on at least six factors: (1) magnitude and rate of virus replication, (2) the fidelity of the viral polymerase, (3) selective pressure or potency of the drug, (4) amount of replication space in the liver, (5) replication fitness of the drug-resistant virus, and (6) genetic barrier of the drug.

Magnitude and Rate of Virus Replication

HBV replication often results in circulating virus concentrations of greater than or equal to 10^8 to 10^{10} virions/mL of plasma in chronically infected patients. Assuming a half-life of 1 day for circulating HBV, more than 10^{11} virions can be produced and cleared per day.[16,17] Bayesian estimates of the evolutionary rate of HBV indicate that the genome can have up to 1 in 10,000 nucleotide substitutions per site per year, and this high substitution rate results in the generation of a vast array of closely related variants or quasispecies.[18] This high substitution rate means that each nucleotide in the genome can be changed every day.

The organization of the HBV genome (see **Fig. 1**) into frame-shifted overlapping ORFs does place some restriction on the final number of viable mutants that can be generated. Indeed, it has been shown that the evolutionary rate of the nonoverlapping regions of the genome is around twofold greater than that of the overlapping regions.[18] The stability of the predominate HBV within the quasispecies pool is maintained by particular selection pressures from the host's innate and adaptive immune system and viability and replication competence of the particular dominant virus isolate.

Fidelity of the Viral Polymerase

Viral mutation rates are generally proportional to the fidelity of their respective polymerases. The substitution rate detected for the HBV genome is approximately

10-fold higher than that for other DNA viruses and more in keeping with the RNA viruses, including the retroviruses.[19,20] The lower mutation rate of most DNA viruses is largely caused by the presence of the proofreading and mismatch repair functions of their polymerase, which is lacking for the polymerases of RNA viruses, retroviruses, and HBV. A consequence of the lower mutation rate in DNA viruses is that longer viral genomes can be replicated and it may be that for HBV the high mutation rate associated with reverse transcription of the pregenomic RNA provides one explanation for it having one of the smallest genomes of all DNA viruses. This lack of proofreading function combined with the high replication rate of HBV also means that genomes that already contain a substitution may acquire a further substitution. Before antiviral therapy, variants carrying single and double mutations potentially associated with drug resistance pre-exist.[21]

Selective Pressure of the Drug

The NAs currently used to treat CHB have previously demonstrated potent activity; however, they are virustatic rather than virucidal and require long-term use. The probability of a mutation associated with drug resistance being selected during therapy depends on the efficacy of that drug; the probability has been depicted graphically as a bell-shaped curve.[22] Hence, a drug with low antiviral activity does not exert significant selection pressure on the virus and the risk of drug resistance emerging is not high. Conversely, complete suppression of viral replication allows almost no opportunity for resistance to emerge because, as highlighted previously, mutagenesis is replication dependent.[21] Because monotherapies exert varying degrees of antiviral activity usually directed at one single target site, they result in the highest probability of selecting for drug resistance. The ideal treatment regimen exerts antiviral activity targeted at different sites in the viral life cycle to reduce significantly the risk of selecting drug-resistant quasispecies. Resistance emerges rapidly when replication occurs in the presence of drug-selection pressure.

Amount of Replication Space in the Liver

Replication space for HBV has been described as the number of liver cells that allow HBV to establish infection[23] or the potential of the liver to accommodate new transcriptional templates or molecules of cccDNA.[24,25] The eventual takeover by a variant virus is dependent on the loss of the original wild-type virus, and is governed by such factors as replication fitness and the turnover and proliferation of hepatocytes.[24,25] Hepatocyte turnover in the normal liver is slow, displaying a typical half-life of over 100 days.[17] This can be reduced to less than 10 days in the setting of increased necroinflammatory activity during direct hepatocyte proliferation, or associated hepatotoxicity.[17] In a fully infected liver, synthesis of new HBV cccDNA molecules can only occur if uninfected cells are generated by normal growth within the liver; hepatocyte proliferation; or loss of wild-type (dominant) cccDNA from existing infected hepatocytes.[26] The precise mechanisms of removal of infected cells is not clear; uninfected hepatocytes may be generated by compensatory proliferation after immune-mediated lysis but noncytopathic curing of HBV cccDNA from infected cells has also been proposed to occur.[27,28]

Replication Fitness of the Drug-resistant Virus

Replication fitness has been defined as the ability to produce offspring in the setting of natural selection.[21] For HBV variants encoding antiviral drug resistance this requires the generation of infectious progeny, dissemination in the liver, and becoming the dominant strain in the presence of the appropriate drug.[23] Replication fitness can only be measured using in vitro coinfection competition assays. Unfortunately, this cannot be conveniently done with HBV because of the lack of a suitable cell culture system that supports complete cycles of viral replication.

Several clinical observations demonstrate the fitness of LMV-resistant HBV. Thibault and colleagues[29] were the first to document the transmissibility of LMV-resistant HBV from patient to patient. Several groups have described the persistence of LMV-resistant HBV as codominant quasispecies with wild-type HBV posttreatment for at least 3 months,[30] or as a minor quasispecies with wild-type HBV posttreatment for almost 1 year.[31]

Genetic Barrier

The genetic barrier of a NA can be considered in terms of the number of substitutions needed for the development of primary antiviral drug resistance. In many instances, resistance to an individual NA can be conferred by a single point mutation. For example, for the L-nucleoside, LMV, and the acyclic phosphonate, ADV, only a single mutation is required to encode for the amino acid changes that confer resistance (substitution of the methionine [M] at position 204 of the rt/polymerase with isoleucine [I], designated rtM204I for LMV and substitution of asparagine [N] at position 236 with threonine [T], designated rtN236T for ADV). For ETV, from the D-cyclopentane group, at least three mutations are required to coexist: (1) rtL180M + rtM204V plus a change at one of rtI169, (2) rtS184, and (3) rtS202 or rtM250. In patients naive to therapy, ETV resistance rarely occurs, even after 5 years of treatment, and resistance is normally found in patients who have already developed LMV-resistant HBV.[32]

In a large heterogeneous viral population, it is likely that variants requiring only a single point mutation to confer resistance pre-exist and with a drug showing low efficacy, these are rapidly selected. A drug that requires the virus to have multiple independent mutations for resistance offers significant advantages because the probability that the appropriate number of pre-existing point mutations occurring by chance decreases as the number of mutations required for resistance increases.

Other Factors

Host factors effecting antiviral therapy include age; previous drug experience; compliance; host genetic factors (eg, inborn errors of metabolism); and the ability efficiently to convert the NA to its active metabolite by intracellular phosphorylation pathways.[33] In addition, there are sequestered sites and sanctuaries of viral replication that may not be accessible to the antiviral agent, such as in the lymphoid system, and the key HBV replicative intermediate, the intrahepatic cccDNA form, is typically recalcitrant to conventional therapy.[34]

PATTERNS AND PATHWAYS OF ANTIVIRAL DRUG RESISTANCE IN CHB
Patterns of Resistance

L-Nucleosides
LMV resistance mutations Antiviral resistance to LMV has been mapped to the tyrosine-methionine-aspartate-aspartate (YMDD) locus in the catalytic or C domain of HBV rt/polymerase (**Table 1**).[34] The primary resistance mutations result in the replacement of the methionine by valine, leucine, or occasionally serine and are designated rtM204I/V/S. Although rtM204I can be found in isolation, M204V/S are only found with other changes, in particular rtL180M (in domain B).[35,36] Other primary mutations that also confer LMV resistance include the substitutions rtA181T/V.[37] Compensatory changes can be found in other domains of the HBV rt/polymerase, such as rtL80V/I,[38] rtV173L,[39] and rtT184S.[40]

Table 1
Patterns and pathways of antiviral drug resistance in chronic hepatitis B in the context of cross-resistance

Pathway	Amino Acid Substitutions in the rt Domain	Lamivudine	Telbivudine	Entecavir	Adefovir	Tenofovir
	Wild-type	S	S	S	S	S
L-Nucleoside (LMV/LdT)	M204I/V	R	R	I	S	S
Acyclic phosphonate (ADV)	N236T	S	S	S	R	I
Shared	A181T/V	I	R	S	R	I
D-Cyclopentane (ETV)	L180M+M204V/I ± I169 ± T184 ± S202 ± M250	R	R	R	S	S

Abbreviations: I, intermediate sensitivity; R, resistant; S, sensitive.

LMV resistance increases progressively during treatment at rates of 14% to 32% annually, exceeding 70% after 48 months of treatment.[10] Factors that increase the risk of development of resistance include high pretherapy serum HBV DNA and ALT levels and the incomplete suppression of viral replication.[10] The main LMV resistance mutations rtM204V/I confer cross-resistance to LdT and the other members that belong to the L-nucleoside structural group (see **Table 1**). Fortunately, these mutations do not confer cross-resistance to ADV or TFV (see **Table 1**), but the rtA181T has been detected during treatment with ADV.[40,41] It is important to note that the rtM204V/I reduces susceptibility to ETV (see **Table 1**).[42]

Mutations that confer LMV resistance decrease in vitro sensitivity to LMV from at least 100-fold to more than 1000-fold. The molecular mechanism of LMV resistance seems to be steric hindrance caused by the β-branched side group of the bulkier valine or isoleucine competing for space with the oxathiolane ring of LMV in the deoxynucleotide triphosphate–binding site (**Fig. 2A**).[43]

LdT resistance mutations LdT is the "unnatural" L-enantiomer of the natural (D-) deoxynucleoside. Structure–activity relationship analysis indicates that the 3′-OH groups of the β-L-2′-deoxynucleosides confer specific antihepadnavirus activity. LdT is efficiently converted into the active triphosphate metabolite and has a long intracellular half-life. The main resistance substitution in the HBV rt/polymerase found with LdT therapy is rtM204I, and this confers to antiviral cross-resistance to LMV (see **Table 1**). Additional specific resistance mutations described include rtA181T/V by the shared pathway (see **Table 1**) and rtL229W/V. Resistance to LdT steadily increased from 4% of prevalent cases at 12 months rising to over 30% after 24 months of monotherapy.

Acyclic phosphonates
ADV resistance mutations Resistance to ADV was initially associated with mutations in the B (rtA181T) and D (N236T) domains of the enzyme.[41,44] HBV resistance to ADV occurs less frequently than resistance to LMV, with a prevalence of around 2% after 2 years, 4% after 3 years, 18% after 4 years, and 29% after 5 years.[45] These ADV-associated mutations in HBV rt/polymerase result in only a modest (threefold to

eightfold) increase in the concentration of the drug required for 50% effective inhibition concentration for viral replication in vitro (EC_{50}), and confer partial cross-resistance to TFV (see **Table 1**), probably because the molecular mechanism of resistance is similar with indirect perturbation of the triphosphate binding site between the A and D domains (see **Fig. 2B**).[43,46] In the case of the rtA181T substitution, this results in an allosteric change affecting the catalytic site of the rt/polymerase (**Table 2**). The rtN236T does not significantly affect sensitivity to LMV,[44] but the rtA181T/V mutations confer partial cross-resistance to LMV (see **Table 1**). Recently, another substitution (rtI233V) has claimed to confer resistance to ADV.[47] In clinical studies, the rtI233V change seems to occur in approximately 2% of all patients with CHB[47,48] but its exact role in ADV failure or nonresponse is yet to be established.

TFV resistance mutations TFV (9-[2-phosphonomethoxypropyl] adenine) is related to ADV and is also a nucleotide acyclic phosphonate. Like ADV, TFV also requires a diphosphorylation process to be converted to its active form. TFV is effective against both HIV and HBV and has been used successfully to treat coinfected patients. TFV, like ADV, is also effective against LMV-resistant virus with rtM204V/I changes. As shown in **Table 1**, the primary mutations associated with ADV resistance (rtA181T/V and/or rtN236T) can decrease the efficacy of TFV.

D-Cyclopentane group

ETV resistance mutations Resistance to ETV was initially described in patients who were already infected with LMV-resistant HBV.[42] Moreover, ETV resistance seems first to require the presence of rtM204V/I (±L180M), followed by the acquisition of other ETV "signature" substitutions in the B domain (rtI169T or rtS184G), C domain (rtS202I), or E domain (rtM250V) of the HBV rt/polymerase. In the absence of the changes associated with LMV resistance, the rtM250V causes an almost 10-fold increase in EC_{50}, whereas the rtT184G and rtS202I changes have little effect.[42,49] In contrast, when the substitutions rtL180M+rtM204V are also present, a greater than 100-fold increase in EC_{50} has been observed. Recently, primary resistance to ETV in a patient naive to NA was reported[50] and required at least three coexisting substitutions to be present, indicating a high genetic barrier for ETV.

The occurrence of resistance to ETV in drug-naive patients is negligible during the first year[51] and remains low (approximately 1%) even after 5 years of treatment.[32] In LMV-experienced patients who were subsequently switched to ETV, however, the frequency of virologic breakthrough was around 50%,[32] limiting the role of ETV salvage therapy in those patients refractory to LMV treatment.

The molecular mechanism of resistance for the rtM250V change is thought to be an alteration of the binding interaction between the DNA primer strand and DNA template strand with the incoming deoxynucleotide triphosphate (see **Fig. 2C**).[52] The mechanism of ETV resistance for the rtT184G+rtS202I is an allosteric change with altered geometry of the nucleotide-binding pocket and DNA template binding of the polymerase (see **Fig. 2D**) near the YMDD site.[52]

Pathways of Resistance

The primary resistance mutations associated with drug failure for CHB are shown in **Fig. 3**. As few as eight substitutions in the HBV polymerase account for primary treatment failure with the currently approved NAs for CHB. Acquisition of primary resistance mutations commits subsequent viral evolution to different pathways.[53]

To date, four pathways have been identified: (1) the L-nucleoside pathway (rtM204V/I), in which LMV and LdT treatment select for rtM204V/I (see **Fig. 3**), which predisposes to subsequent ETV resistance; (2) the acyclic phosphonate pathway (rtN236T) in which ADV and TFV treatment select for or consolidate rtN236T[44,54]; (3) a shared pathway (rtA181T/V) whereby treatment with either L-nucleosides or acyclic phosphonates can result in selection of rtA181T/V, which occurs in about 40% of cases of ADV failure but less than 5% of cases of LMV failure[55]; and (4) the D-cyclopentane or

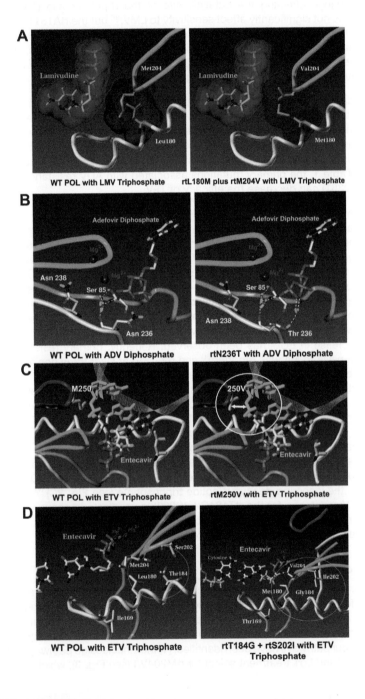

A

WT POL with LMV Triphosphate   rtL180M plus rtM204V with LMV Triphosphate

B

WT POL with ADV Diphosphate   rtN236T with ADV Diphosphate

C

WT POL with ETV Triphosphate   rtM250V with ETV Triphosphate

D

WT POL with ETV Triphosphate   rtT184G + rtS202I with ETV Triphosphate

Table 2
Proposed molecular mechanisms of antiviral drug resistance in the HBV polymerase

Antiviral	Mutation	Proposed Mechanism
LMV/LdT	rtM204I/V	Catalytic site: allosteric change/ steric hindrance
ADV(1)	rtN236T	Triphosphate binding site: allosteric change
ADV (2)	rtA181T/V	Catalytic site: allosteric change
ETV (1)	rtM250V[a]	Primer binding site: allosteric change
ETV (2)	rtT184G+ rtS202I[a]	Catalytic site: allosteric change

[a] Plus LMV resistance at rtM204V + rtL180M.

ETV-naive resistance pathway (rtM204V/I ± rtL180M and one or more substitutions at rtI169, rtT184, S202, or M250). Three substitutions are required to coexist, accounting for the very low resistance profile of ETV (see **Table 1**).[50]

The pathway concept has been proposed as a guide to assist physicians with the long-term management of patients with CHB.[53] In the HIV-antiretroviral arena, this approach has been extended into "antiretroviral drug sequencing," which refers to the preferred use of a particular NA in initial therapy based on the assumption that virologic failure and drug resistance might later develop and be overcome by the introduction of a sequential drug (in combination).[56] The overall concept is that treatment sequencing (ie, a defined treatment using a sequence of drugs) provides an effective strategy to cope with virologic failure. The primary objectives are the avoidance of accumulation of mutations and the selection of multidrug resistant (MDR) viruses. In CHB, where very-long-term therapies are necessary to ensure adequate virologic

Fig. 2. (A) Lamivudine resistance. The figure illustrates effect of changes that confer LMV resistance. LMV triphosphate is shown in the binding pocket. The bulkier valine of rtM204V competes for space with the oxathiolane group of LMV resulting in steric hindrance. (*Data from* Bartholomeusz A, Tehan BG, Chalmers DK. Comparisons of the HBV and HIV polymerase, and antiviral resistance mutations. Antivir Ther 2004;9:149.) (B) Adefovir resistance. The rtN236T substitution causes indirect perturbation of the triphosphate binding site and alteration of the Mg 2+ binding site. (*Data from* Bartholomeusz A, Locarnini S, Ayres A, et al. Molecular modelling of hepatitis B virus polymerase and adefovir resistance identifies three clusters of mutations. Hepatology 2004;40:246A; and Bartholomeusz A, Tehan BG, Chalmers DK. Comparisons of the HBV and HIV polymerase, and antiviral resistance mutations. Antivir Ther 2004;9:149.) (C) Entecavir resistance. This figure shows how the M250 interacts with the primer strand (*left*) whereas the M250V substitution alters the binding interaction between the primer stand and the incoming dNTP (*right*). (*Data from* Warner N, Locarnini S, Colledge D, et al. Molecular modelling of entecavir resistant mutations in the hepatitis B virus polymerase selected during therapy. Hepatology 2004;40:245A.) (D) Entecavir resistance. This figure shows how the wild-type rtT184 and rtS202 stabilize the interaction between the B and C domains (*left*) and how with the resistance substitutions rtT184G and rtS202I these result in an altered geometry of the nucleotide binding pocket (*right*). (*Data from* Warner N, Locarnini S, Colledge D, et al. Molecular modelling of entecavir resistant mutations in the hepatitis B virus polymerase selected during therapy. Hepatology 2004;40:245A.)

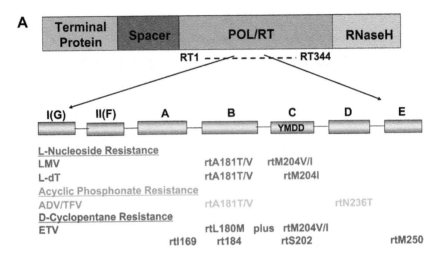

Fig. 3. (A) The primary antiviral drug-resistance associated changes and evolutionary pathways.[53] This and the other three pathways are described in detail in the text. (B) Antiviral drug-resistance associated changes in the HBV polymerase and evolutionary pathways.

suppression, the clinician should ask: "If I start with drug A, what options will be available after 1 year, 3 years, or 5 years if resistance develops?"

Cross-resistance

Cross resistance is defined as resistance to drugs to which a virus has never been exposed as a result of changes that have been selected for by the use of another drug (see **Table 1**).[57] The resistance-associated mutations selected by a particular NA confer at least some degree of cross-resistance to other members of its structural group but may also diminish the sensitivity to NAs from other groups.[36] The initial drug choice and subsequent rescue therapies should be based on a knowledge of cross-resistance,[58] so that the second agent has a different resistance profile to the failing agent.[8,9] The advantage of using the add-on combination approach of NAs with complementary cross-resistance profiles has recently been highlighted[8,9,58] and a summary of cross-resistance profiles based on the viral resistance "pathways" approach is shown in **Table 1**.

Multidrug Resistance

Monotherapy can promote selection for MDR strains of HBV, especially when patients are treated sequentially with drugs with overlapping resistance profiles, such as with LMV followed by ETV[59,60] or LMV followed by ADV.[61,62] Clonal analyses have shown that MDR usually occurs by the sequential acquisition of resistance mutations by the same viral genome; mutants that arise from this selection process may have full resistance to multiple drugs. Studies have shown that MDR strains arise if an "add-on" therapeutic strategy does not result in rapid viral suppression, particularly if there is sufficient replication space available for the mutants to spread (ie, necroinflammatory activity indicated by high levels of serum ALT, resulting in hepatocyte proliferation). A detailed analysis of variants in a patient with an MDR strain of HBV after liver transplantation revealed mutations in the overlapping P and S genes that conferred resistance to LMV and ADV and a decreased recognition of the virus by anti-HBs antibodies.[62] These findings emphasize the need to achieve complete viral suppression during antiviral therapy.

A specific single amino acid substitution may confer MDR (see **Table 1**). This was shown with the rtA181V/T substitution, which is responsible not only for decreased susceptibility to the L-nucleosides LMV and LdT but also to the acyclic phosphonates ADV and TFV.[55,63] This highlights the potential usefulness of genotypic testing in patients with treatment failure to determine the viral resistance mutation profile and thereby tailor therapy to the major viral strain circulating (**Fig. 4**). Studies of the HIV response to antiretrovirals have shown that drug resistance testing can be used to monitor response to therapy and aid in the selection of new drug regimens for patients who have failed to respond.[57]

CONSEQUENCES OF DRUG RESISTANCE
Impact on Disease Severity

Following the development of drug resistance, there is an increase in viral load and consequent increase in serum ALT levels several weeks to months later, which in time may manifest as progressive liver disease.[10,11,15] In patients refractory to L-nucleoside therapy, the risk of increased serum ALT levels is usually temporally correlated with the establishment of resistant virus.[64] Such patients may also be at risk of an ALT flare, which may be accompanied by hepatic decompensation if there is underlying cirrhosis.[64] The emergence of LMV-resistant variants and their association with adverse consequences for liver disease has been demonstrated histologically.[65] Furthermore, in the setting of cirrhosis, patients successfully treated with LMV who maintained wild-type virus had a significantly lower risk of liver disease progression compared with those who received placebo, but this effect was lost in patients who developed LMV-resistant HBV.[66]

Polymerase-Surface Gene Overlap

As shown in **Fig. 1**, the S gene, encoding HBsAg, is completely contained with the P gene, although in a different reading frame. This gene overlap is important because it has been shown that the common mutations encoding the substitutions causing LMV resistance (eg, rtV173L + rtL180M + rtM204V), can result in concomitant nucleotide changes encoding important and significant changes in HBsAg (surface [s]E164D + sI195M), which substantially reduce anti-HBs (vaccine-associated) binding in vitro.[67] Likewise, in adefovir failure, the rtA181T substitution can be found either by itself or in association with rtN236T, in up to 40% of cases. The mutation encoding the rtA181T results in a sW172[STOP] in the overlapping HBsAg. This HBV variant has

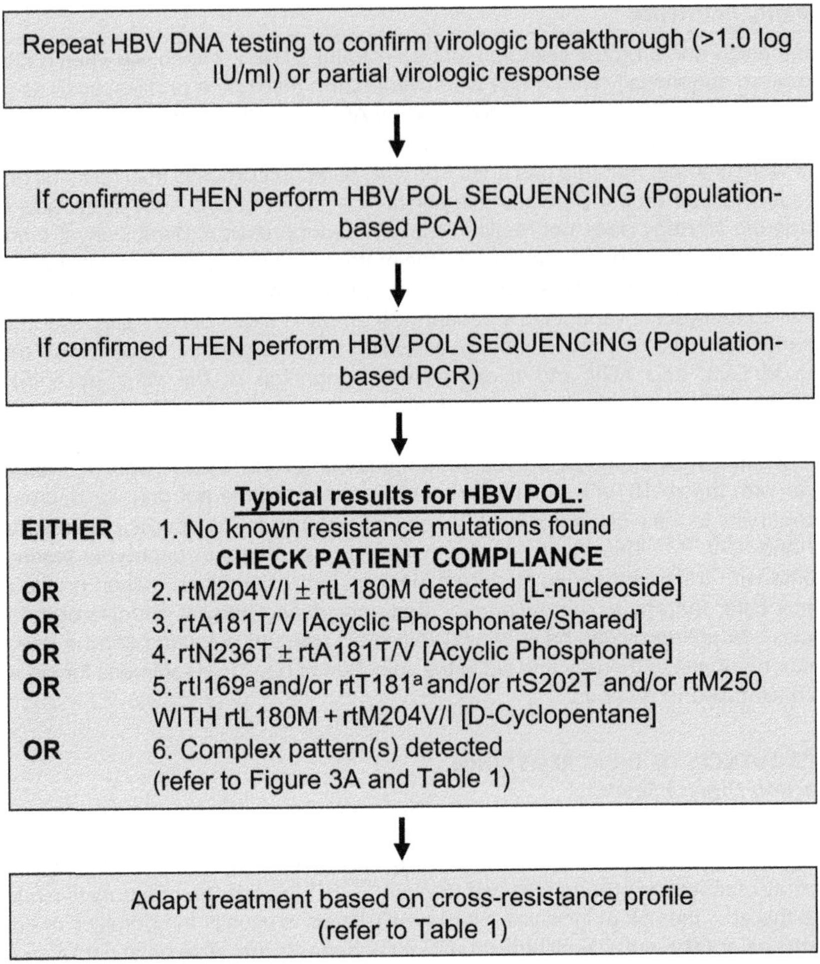

Repeat HBV DNA testing to confirm virologic breakthrough (>1.0 log IU/ml) or partial virologic response

If confirmed THEN perform HBV POL SEQUENCING (Population-based PCA)

If confirmed THEN perform HBV POL SEQUENCING (Population-based PCR)

↓

Typical results for HBV POL:

EITHER	1. No known resistance mutations found **CHECK PATIENT COMPLIANCE**
OR	2. rtM204V/I ± rtL180M detected [L-nucleoside]
OR	3. rtA181T/V [Acyclic Phosphonate/Shared]
OR	4. rtN236T ± rtA181T/V [Acyclic Phosphonate]
OR	5. rtI169[a] and/or rtT181[a] and/or rtS202T and/or rtM250 WITH rtL180M + rtM204V/I [D-Cyclopentane]
OR	6. Complex pattern(s) detected (refer to Figure 3A and Table 1)

Adapt treatment based on cross-resistance profile (refer to Table 1)

Fig. 4. Proposed management flow chart for the first virologic breakthrough or partial virologic response in a patient with CHB undergoing NA therapy. The codons associated with ETV resistance (#) are described in the text. (*Adapted from* Zoulim F, Locarnini S. Hepatitis B virus resistance to nucleos(t)ide analogs. Gastroenterology 2009;137:1593; with permission.)

been shown to be defective in virion secretion,[55] retained in the cell, and to behave as a dominant negative mutant for wild-type HBV secretion. The clinical implication of these observations is that the virologic case definition of drug resistance of greater than 1 $\log_{10}$ IU/mL from nadir in two consecutive samples taken 1 month apart[7–9] may not be appropriate if this mutant is (co)-selected. The viral load, following first appearance of rtA181T, only very gradually increases from nadir over 12 months. The truncated surface proteins expressed from this variant have also been implicated in enhancing the progression to hepatocellular carcinoma.[68] These observations again highlight the value of HBV P gene sequence analysis and HBV viral load monitoring in patients undergoing antiviral therapy.

Public Health Relevance of Resistance

The in vitro studies of the overlap between the P and S genes, which showed reduced anti-HBs binding for variants with LMV resistance, have now been extended to in vivo analyses. The common LMV-resistant mutant (rtV173L + rtL180M + rtM204V), which encodes the surface changes sE164D + sI195M in HBsAg, was infectious in hepatitis B immunized chimpanzees that had high titers of circulating anti-HBs prechallenge.[69] The chimpanzee HBV transmission study also established the genetic stability of the HBV rtV173L + rtL180M + rtM204V variant in a nonimmunized chimpanzee, in which no reversion to wild-type was detected compared with infection with the sG145R vaccine escape mutant, which quickly reverted to wild-type.[69] This latter observation demonstrates the important role of compensatory mutations in "fixing the genetic archive," especially in the setting of transmission of virus with NA resistance.

Transmission of Antiviral Drug-resistant HBV

The clinical evidence for the spread or transmission of LMV-resistant HBV has to date been limited. It was first reported in conjunction with concomitant HIV infection[29] where a patient with HIV infection undergoing antiviral therapy, which included LMV, later developed primary infection with an LMV-resistant HBV. Similar LMV-resistant mutations have also been found in the HBV isolated from dialysis patients with occult HBV infection.[70] These dialysis patients were not undergoing antiviral therapy, yet 50% of the patients with occult HBV infection were found to have LMV-resistant virus. Furthermore, LMV-resistant HBV has been detected in asymptomatic chronically infected individuals not yet commenced on LMV therapy.[71] Very recently, Hayashi and colleagues[72] have identified two cases of LMV-resistant HBV associated with acute hepatitis B out of a screening population of 45 inpatients admitted with serologically confirmed acute hepatitis. Both patients were male and infected with the rtL180M + rtM204V/I variants, and seemed to have acquired HBV sexually, one case by heterosexual (from a female prostitute) and the other by male-to-male transmission.

The transmission of LMV-resistant HBV has important implications for the control of HBV infection, especially at the global level. The main strategy of the World Health Organization is centered on primary prevention through vaccination.

Unfortunately, the prevalence of NA-resistant HBV is becoming more widespread. LMV resistance, in particular, has become a problem in the Asia-Pacific region because the drug is often the cheapest treatment option. Furthermore, many patients are maintained on LMV monotherapy even after the emergence of drug resistance, and this may result in the acquisition of more compensatory mutations that increase the chance of fixation and persistence of the corresponding HBV cccDNA in the patient's liver.[73] This further complicates the public health challenge of drug resistance because not only could variant virus be transmitted to nonimmunized individuals,[29,72] but a subpopulation of variants have the potential to infect immunized individuals.[69] In such cases, neutralizing antibodies (anti-HBs) would provide selection pressure that would enrich for drug-resistant HBV strains over wild-type virus,[74] thereby establishing these strains more widely in the community.

PREVENTION OF DRUG RESISTANCE

The spread of drug-resistant HBV can be reduced by avoiding unnecessary drug use, choosing drugs and combinations more carefully, and continually monitoring or performing targeted surveillance for drug resistance.[21] Because of the unusual replication strategy of HBV, viral populations are genetically heterogeneous, so that even treatment-naive patients have pre-existing minor populations encoding resistance in the absence of selection pressure from antiviral drugs. Most patients may not require antiviral therapy. Several professional bodies (including the American Association for the Study of the Liver, the European Association for the Study of the Liver, the Asian Pacific Association for the Study of the Liver, and the National Institutes of Health) publish regularly updated guidelines to assist clinicians with recognition, diagnosis, prevention, and management of CHB. These are unanimous in recommending that therapy should be considered for patients with only more active or advanced liver disease and others most likely to respond in the context of defined treatment end points. Treatment algorithms have been developed to assist in identification of suitable candidates for treatment and to determine when to initiate treatment.

Because drug-resistant HBV quasispecies are established and expand through replication, antiviral therapy, once initiated, should aim to suppress viral replication as completely and rapidly as possible. The lower risk of resistance developing to TFV and ETV (compared with LMV, LdT, and ADV) supports their use as first-line therapy generally and in particular for HBV-infected patients who have received liver transplants and those with advanced liver disease, because development of drug resistance is more likely to precipitate clinical deterioration in these groups.

Combination chemotherapy is being used more frequently to treat CHB. It is effective when the appropriate combinations are used and can reduce the risk of drug resistance.[75] Although HBV mutants that are resistant to single drugs may exist before therapy starts and can evolve rapidly in patients, HBV mutants with MDR are much less likely to exist before treatment. Even though NAs target the same viral enzyme, the resistance profiles of NAs from each structural group show that there are sufficient differences in their mode of action for combination therapy to decrease the risk of emerging resistance. Combination therapy using NAs with a complementary cross-resistance profile minimizes the development of resistance but unfortunately does not seem to increase antiviral efficacy compared with single-drug therapy.[75,76] Use of an immunomodulatory agent, such as interferon, with an NA that has direct antiviral activity seems to be a logical approach for combination therapy. Although initial clinical trials of such combinations using predominantly LMV as the NA have been disappointing, results from later trials are more encouraging. The added benefit of the combination tends to be lost, however, after treatment cessation.[77,78] It may be that combination therapy of pegylated interferon with the more potent drugs, such as ETV and TFV, may have greater efficacy.

Each patient's response to treatment should be monitored carefully so that drug resistance can be detected early, before viral breakthrough and disease progression. Assays for serum levels of HBV DNA and ALT should be performed 3 to 6 months after commencement of therapy to check for efficacy and compliance; lack of compliance is the most common cause of primary treatment failure. Additional testing, performed at 6 monthly intervals during the first 2 years of treatment, is recommended for patients with mild liver disease. Patients should then be assessed by measuring viral load and ALT levels every 3 to 6 months for the next 2 years of therapy; this is the time in which the probability of developing resistance increases. The potential life-threatening consequences of the emergence of resistance may manifest more rapidly in patients with advanced disease; these patients should be tested for viral load and have ALT levels monitored every 3 months. If the viral load increases by greater than 1 $\log_{10}$ IU/mL, sequencing of the P gene should be considered to identify resistance mutations and determine the optimal therapeutic approach, based on cross-resistance profiles (see **Fig. 4** and **Table 1**).

MANAGEMENT OF DRUG RESISTANCE

The management of NA drug resistance has been recently updated in the European Association for the Study of the Liver Clinical Practice Guidelines[58] and reviewed by Zoulim and Locarnini.[73] Virologic breakthrough in compliant patients is typically associated with the emergence of viral resistance. Resistance is associated with prior treatment with NAs or, in treatment-naive patients, with high baseline levels of HBV DNA, a slow decline in HBV DNA levels, and partial virologic response to treatment. Resistance should be identified as early as possible, before ALT levels increase, by monitoring HBV DNA levels and if possible identifying the NA resistance profile; the therapeutic strategy to be adopted can be determined based on this information. Clinical and virology studies have demonstrated the benefit of an early (as soon as viral load increases) modification of treatment.[58,79,80] In cases of resistance, an appropriate rescue therapy should be initiated that has the most effective antiviral effect and minimal risk for selection of MDR strains. Adding a second drug that is not in the same cross-resistance group as the initial NA is the recommended strategy.

Table 1 shows the cross-resistance data for the most frequent resistant HBV variants.[58,81] Treatment adaptation should be performed accordingly and is summarized in **Box 1**[73]:

Note that the safety of some combinations in the longer term is presently unknown and that add-on therapy is not always successful in achieving adequate viral inhibition (ie, HBV DNA not detected by sensitive real-time polymerase chain reaction assay).

In HIV infection, drug-resistant virus can be transmitted by sexual, parenteral, and perinatal exposures, and has been found in up to 20% of incident cases.[82] In such instances, initial antiretroviral treatment options may be limited and the virologic response compromised in those patients.[83] As a consequence, routine drug resistance testing has recently been recommended for all newly diagnosed HIV-infected individuals, with the assumption that transmitted drug-resistant virus persists for an unknown period of time after infection.[84] Little and colleagues[85] have recently demonstrated that following transmission of drug-resistant HIV, patients typically show a transient high-titer viremia, followed by a spontaneous decline to a steady state or new "set-point" viremia. During these first 4 to 6 months, polymerase chain reaction–based sequencing of plasma virus typically detects only resistant virus. In subsequent years, it has been observed that there is a gradual process of random and potentially selective mutations that result in the appearance of genetic mixtures of HIV at the sites of previous drug-resistant mutations. This is then followed by ultimate replacement

---

Box 1
Treatment adaptation

- LMV resistance: add TFV (add ADV if TFV not available).

- ADV resistance: it is recommended to switch to TFV if available and add a second drug without cross-resistance. If an rtN236T substitution is present, add LMV, ETV, or LdT or switch to TFV plus emtricitabine. If an rtA181V/T substitution is present, it is recommended to add-on ETV or to switch to TFV plus ETV or TFV plus emtricitabine (as a single tablet: Truvada).

- LdT resistance: it is recommended to add TFV (or ADV if TFV is not available).

- ETV resistance: it is recommended to add TFV.

- TFV resistance: primary resistance to TFV has not been confirmed to date. It is recommended that genotyping and phenotyping be done by a reference-type laboratory to determine the cross-resistance profile. ETV, LdT, LMV, or emtricitabine could be added but depend on the resistance profile (see **Table 1**).

with wild-type virus. It is important to note, however, that the resistant variants persist for the life of the patient, harbored within the reservoir of long-lived memory CD-4 cells. This scenario in HIV has particular relevance and implications for the World Health Organization program for the control of hepatitis B by vaccination[74] and the current widespread use of low genetic barrier and potency drugs, such as LMV, in medium-to-high HBV prevalence countries.

SUMMARY

The current emerging patterns of antiviral drug resistance mapped to the HBV rt/polymerase are complex. The eight substitutions associated with primary drug resistance fall into four major pathways, however, which seem reasonably predictable based on analysis. Nevertheless, broad clusters of compensatory mutations, especially during LMV therapy, are compromising future salvage therapy options. Algorithms for the use of viral load and HBV genotyping and P gene sequencing clearly need to be developed for patients receiving NA therapy.[7-9] There is also a strong need for the availability and more widespread use of interactive database programs to guide rescue therapy in CHB.[86] The unique genetic arrangement of the HBV genome with the P and S genes overlapping (see **Fig. 1**) has substantial public health and diagnostic implications because of the ability of emerging drug resistance changes modifying HBsAg.[55,67] Some of these concomitant HBsAg changes may even have oncogenic potential because truncated surface proteins have been associated with the development of hepatocellular carcinoma.[68]

Clearly, resistance to hepatitis B therapies must be prevented by prescribing NAs with high potency and a high genetic barrier to resistance (ETV or TFV) and ensuring patient compliance and monitoring the effectiveness of patient treatment with the goals of therapy being appropriately controlled HBV replication.[58] Because "no replication equals no resistance" under most circumstances, this must become an important mantra for treating physicians and the end point of therapy for the patient. In this way, the possible catastrophic public health risks and consequences of emergence of drug resistance linked to vaccine escape should likewise be eliminated. Clinical experience to date with less potent NAs as monotherapy has shown the limitations of this approach and has provided a strong case that for long-term suppression of viral replication combination chemotherapy is required. Provided that appropriate combinations of agents with complementary resistance profiles and a high genetic barrier of resistance are used, such approaches should arrest disease progression by a consistent reduction of viral load and consequent reduced risk of the emergence of drug resistance. It is not known whether an end point of undetectable viremia can provide other benefits, such as HBeAg seroconversion,[87] and whether sustained virologic suppression with histologic improvement could result in HBsAg seroconversion. A reasonable clinical goal, however, is the application of this concept by the optimization of combination therapies analogous to highly active antiretroviral therapy for people infected with HIV.[88]

REFERENCES

1. Locarnini S. Molecular virology and the development of resistant mutants: implications for therapy. Semin Liver Dis 2005;25(Suppl 1):9.
2. Chisari FV, Ferrari C. Hepatitis B virus immunopathogenesis. Annu Rev Immunol 1995;13:29
3. Chen CJ, Yang HI, Su J, et al. Risk of hepatocellular carcinoma across a biological gradient of serum hepatitis B virus DNA level. JAMA 2006;295:65.

4. Iloeje UH, Yang HI, Su J, et al. Predicting cirrhosis risk based on the level of circulating hepatitis B viral load. Gastroenterology 2006;130:678.

5. Shaw T, Locarnini S. Entecavir for the treatment of chronic hepatitis B. Expert Rev Anti Infect Ther 2004;2:853.

6. Domingo E. Quasispecies and the development of new antiviral strategies. Prog Drug Res 2003;60:133.

7. Locarnini S, Hatzakis A, Heathcote J, et al. Management of antiviral resistance in patients with chronic hepatitis B. Antivir Ther 2004;9:679.

8. Lok AS, Zoulim F, Locarnini S, et al. Antiviral drug-resistant HBV: standardization of nomenclature and assays and recommendations for management. Hepatology 2007;46:254.

9. Pawlotsky JM, Dusheiko G, Hatzakis A, et al. Virologic monitoring of hepatitis B virus therapy in clinical trials and practice: recommendations for a standardized approach. Gastroenterology 2008;134:405.

10. Lai CL, Dienstag J, Schiff E, et al. Prevalence and clinical correlates of YMDD variants during lamivudine therapy for patients with chronic hepatitis B. Clin Infect Dis 2003;36:687.

11. Nafa S, Ahmed S, Tavan D, et al. Early detection of viral resistance by determination of hepatitis B virus polymerase mutations in patients treated by lamivudine for chronic hepatitis B. Hepatology 2000;32:1078.

12. Zoulim F, Poynard T, Degos F, et al. A prospective study of the evolution of lamivudine resistance mutations in patients with chronic hepatitis B treated with lamivudine. J Viral Hepat 2006;13:278.

13. Hadziyannis SJ, Tassopoulos NC, Heathcote EJ, et al. Long-term therapy with adefovir dipivoxil for HBeAg-negative chronic hepatitis B for up to 5 years. Gastroenterology 2006;131:1743.

14. Lai CL, Gane E, Liaw YF, et al. Telbivudine versus lamivudine in patients with chronic hepatitis B. N Engl J Med 2007;357:2576.

15. Yuen MF, Sablon E, Hui CK, et al. Factors associated with hepatitis B virus DNA breakthrough in patients receiving prolonged lamivudine therapy. Hepatology 2001;34:785.

16. Lewin SR, Ribeiro RM, Walters T, et al. Analysis of hepatitis B viral load decline under potent therapy: complex decay profiles observed. Hepatology 2001;34:1012.

17. Nowak MA, Bonhoeffer S, Hill AM, et al. Viral dynamics in hepatitis B virus infection. Proc Natl Acad Sci U S A 1996;93:4398.

18. Zhou Y, Holmes EC. Bayesian estimates of the evolutionary rate and age of hepatitis B virus. J Mol Evol 2007;65:197.

19. Duffy S, Shackelton LA, Holmes EC. Rates of evolutionary change in viruses: patterns and determinants. Nat Rev Genet 2008;9:267.

20. Girones R, Miller RH. Mutation rate of the hepadnavirus genome. Virology 1989; 170:595.

21. Richman DD. The impact of drug resistance on the effectiveness of chemotherapy for chronic hepatitis B. Hepatology 2000;32:866.

22. Richman DD. The implications of drug resistance for strategies of combination antiviral chemotherapy. Antiviral Res 1996;29:31.

23. Villet S, Billioud G, Pichoud C, et al. In vitro characterization of viral fitness of therapy-resistant hepatitis B variants. Gastroenterology 2009;136:168.

24. Zhang YY, Summers J. Enrichment of a precore-minus mutant of duck hepatitis B virus in experimental mixed infections. J Virol 1999;73:3616.

25. Zhang YY, Summers J. Low dynamic state of viral competition in a chronic avian hepadnavirus infection. J Virol 2000;74:5257.

26. Seeger C, Mason WS. Hepatitis B virus biology. Microbiol Mol Biol Rev 2000;64:51.
27. Mason WS, Jilbert AR, Summers J. Clonal expansion of hepatocytes during chronic woodchuck hepatitis virus infection. Proc Natl Acad Sci U S A 2005; 102:1139.
28. Mason WS, Litwin S, Xu C, et al. Hepatocyte turnover in transient and chronic hepadnavirus infections. J Viral Hepat 2007;14(Suppl 1):22.
29. Thibault V, Aubron-Olivier C, Agut H, et al. Primary infection with a lamivudine-resistant hepatitis B virus. AIDS 2002;16:131.
30. Niesters HG, De Man RA, Pas SD, et al. Identification of a new variant in the YMDD motif of the hepatitis B virus polymerase gene selected during lamivudine therapy. J Med Microbiol 2002;51:695.
31. Lok AS, Zoulim F, Locarnini S, et al. Monitoring drug resistance in chronic hepatitis B virus (HBV)-infected patients during lamivudine therapy: evaluation of performance of INNO-LiPA HBV DR assay. J Clin Microbiol 2002;40:3729.
32. Tenney DJ, Rose RE, Baldick CJ, et al. Long-term monitoring shows hepatitis B virus resistance to entecavir in nucleoside-naive patients is rare through 5 years of therapy. Hepatology 2009;49:1503.
33. Shaw T, Locarnini SA. Preclinical aspects of lamivudine and famciclovir against hepatitis B virus. J Viral Hepat 1999;6:89.
34. Locarnini S, Mason WS. Cellular and virological mechanisms of HBV drug resistance. J Hepatol 2006;44:422.
35. Delaney WE, Locarnini S, Shaw T. Resistance of hepatitis B virus to antiviral drugs: current aspects and directions for future investigation. Antivir Chem Chemother 2001;12:1.
36. Shaw T, Bartholomeusz A, Locarnini S. HBV drug resistance: mechanisms, detection and interpretation. J Hepatol 2006;44:593.
37. Yeh CT, Chien RN, Chu CM, et al. Clearance of the original hepatitis B virus YMDD-motif mutants with emergence of distinct lamivudine-resistant mutants during prolonged lamivudine therapy. Hepatology 2000;31:1318.
38. Ogata N, Fujii K, Takigawa S, et al. Novel patterns of amino acid mutations in the hepatitis B virus polymerase in association with resistance to lamivudine therapy in japanese patients with chronic hepatitis B. J Med Virol 1999;59:270.
39. Delaney WE, Yang H, Westland CE, et al. The hepatitis B virus polymerase mutation rtV173L is selected during lamivudine therapy and enhances viral replication in vitro. J Virol 2003;77:11833.
40. Bartholomeusz A, Locarnini S, Ayres A, et al. Mechanistic basis for hepatitis B virus resistance to acyclic nucleoside phosphonate analogues, adefovir and tenofovir. Hepatology 2005;42(Suppl 1):594A.
41. Fung SK, Andreone P, Han SH, et al. Adefovir-resistant hepatitis B can be associated with viral rebound and hepatic decompensation. J Hepatol 2005;43:937.
42. Tenney DJ, Levine SM, Rose RE, et al. Clinical emergence of entecavir-resistant hepatitis B virus requires additional substitutions in virus already resistant to Lamivudine. Antimicrob Agents Chemother 2004;48:3498.
43. Bartholomeusz A, Tehan BG, Chalmers DK. Comparisons of the HBV and HIV polymerase, and antiviral resistance mutations. Antivir Ther 2004;9:149.
44. Angus P, Vaughan R, Xiong S, et al. Resistance to adefovir dipivoxil therapy associated with the selection of a novel mutation in the HBV polymerase. Gastroenterology 2003;125:292.
45. Hadziyannis SJ, Tassopoulos NC, Heathcote EJ, et al. Long-term therapy with adefovir dipivoxil for HBeAg-negative chronic hepatitis B. N Engl J Med 2005; 352:2673.

46. Bartholomeusz A, Locarnini S, Ayres A, et al. Molecular modelling of hepatitis b virus polymerase and adefovir resistance identifies three clusters of mutations. Hepatology 2004;40(Suppl 1):246A.

47. Schildgen O, Sirma H, Funk A, et al. Variant of hepatitis B virus with primary resistance to adefovir. N Engl J Med 2006;354:1807.

48. Chang TT, Lai CL. Hepatitis B virus with primary resistance to adefovir. N Engl J Med 2006;355:322.

49. Levine S, Hernandez D, Yamanaka G, et al. Efficacies of entecavir against lamivudine-resistant hepatitis B virus replication and recombinant polymerases in vitro. Antimicrob Agents Chemother 2002;46:2525.

50. Suzuki F, Akuta N, Suzuki Y, et al. Selection of a virus strain resistant to entecavir in a nucleoside-naive patient with hepatitis B of genotype H. J Clin Virol 2007;39:149.

51. Colonno RJ, Rose R, Baldick CJ, et al. Entecavir resistance is rare in nucleoside naive patients with hepatitis B. Hepatology 2006;44:1656.

52. Warner N, Locarnini S, Colledge D, et al. Molecular modelling of entecavir resistant mutations in the hepatitis B virus polymerase selected during therapy. Hepatology 2004;40:245A.

53. Yuen L, Bartholomeusz A, Ayres A, et al. Multidrug resistance and cross-resistance pathways in HBV as a consequence of treatment failure [abstract #949]. Hepatology 2007;46(4 Suppl 1):659A.

54. Van Bommel F, Trojan J, Wasmuth H, et al. Efficacy of tenofovir DF for the treatment of adefovir resistance [abstract 960]. Hepatology 2007;46(Suppl 1):664A.

55. Warner N, Locarnini S. The antiviral drug selected hepatitis B virus rtA181T/sW172∗ mutant has a dominant negative secretion defect and alters the typical profile of viral rebound. Hepatology 2008;48:88.

56. Martinez-Cajas JL, Wainberg MA. Antiretroviral therapy: optimal sequencing of therapy to avoid resistance. Drugs 2008;68:43.

57. Clavel F, Hance AJ. HIV drug resistance. N Engl J Med 2004;350:1023.

58. EASL Clinical Practice Guidelines. Management of chronic hepatitis B. Hepatology 2009;50:227.

59. Villet S, Ollivet A, Pichoud C, et al. Stepwise process for the development of entecavir resistance in a chronic hepatitis B virus infected patient. J Hepatol 2007; 46:531.

60. Yim HJ, Hussain M, Liu Y, et al. Evolution of multi-drug resistant hepatitis B virus during sequential therapy. Hepatology 2006;44:703.

61. Brunelle MN, Jacquard AC, Pichoud C, et al. Susceptibility to antivirals of a human HBV strain with mutations conferring resistance to both lamivudine and adefovir. Hepatology 2005;41:1391.

62. Villet S, Pichoud C, Villeneuve JP, et al. Selection of a multiple drug-resistant hepatitis B virus strain in a liver-transplanted patient. Gastroenterology 2006; 131:1253.

63. Villet S, Pichoud C, Billioud G, et al. Impact of hepatitis B virus rtA181V/T mutants on hepatitis B treatment failure. J Hepatol 2008;48:747.

64. Lok AS, Lai CL, Leung N, et al. Long-term safety of lamivudine treatment in patients with chronic hepatitis B. Gastroenterology 2003;125:1714.

65. Dienstag JL, Goldin RD, Heathcote EJ, et al. Histological outcome during long-term lamivudine therapy. Gastroenterology 2003;124:105.

66. Liaw YF, Sung JJ, Chow WC, et al. Lamivudine for patients with chronic hepatitis B and advanced liver disease. N Engl J Med 2004;351:1521.

67. Torresi J, Earnest-Silveira L, Deliyannis G, et al. Reduced antigenicity of the hepatitis B virus HBsAg protein arising as a consequence of sequence changes in the

overlapping polymerase gene that are selected by lamivudine therapy. Virology 2002;293:305.

68. Lai MW, Huang SF, Hsu CW, et al. Identification of nonsense mutations in hepatitis B virus S gene in patients with hepatocellular carcinoma developed after lamivudine therapy. Antivir Ther 2009;14:249.

69. Kamili S, Sozzi V, Thompson G, et al. Efficacy of hepatitis B vaccine against antiviral drug-resistant hepatitis B virus mutants in the chimpanzee model. Hepatology 2009;49:1483.

70. Besisik F, Karaca C, Akyuz F, et al. Occult HBV infection and YMDD variants in hemodialysis patients with chronic HCV infection. J Hepatol 2003;38:506.

71. Kobayashi S, Ide T, Sata M. Detection of YMDD motif mutations in some lamivudine-untreated asymptomatic hepatitis B virus carriers. J Hepatol 2001; 34:584.

72. Hayashi K, Katano Y, Ishigami M, et al. Prevalence and clinical characterization of patients with acute hepatitis B induced by lamivudine-resistantstrains. J Gastroenterol Hepatol 2010;25:745–9.

73. Zoulim F, Locarnini S. Hepatitis B virus resistance to nucleos(t)ide analogues. Gastroenterology 2009;137:1593.

74. Clements C, Coghlan B, Creati M, et al. Global control of hepatitis B infection: does the potential for antigenic change of the virus in the face of antiviral treatment affect the global hepatitis B immunization programme? Bull World Health Organ 2009;88(1):1–80.

75. Bowden S, Shaw T, Hepatitis B. The case for combination therapy. Curr Opin Investig Drugs 2009;10:795.

76. Sung JJ, Lai JY, Zeuzem S, et al. Lamivudine compared with lamivudine and adefovir dipivoxil for the treatment of HBeAg-positive chronic hepatitis B. J Hepatol 2008;48:728.

77. Lau GK, Piratvisuth T, Luo KX, et al. Peginterferon Alfa-2a, lamivudine, and the combination for HBeAg-positive chronic hepatitis B. N Engl J Med 2005;352: 2682.

78. Marcellin P, Lau GK, Bonino F, et al. Peginterferon alfa-2a alone, lamivudine alone, and the two in combination in patients with HBeAg-negative chronic hepatitis B. N Engl J Med 2004;351:1206.

79. Lampertico P, Vigano M, Manenti E, et al. Low resistance to adefovir combined with lamivudine: a 3-year study of 145 lamivudine-resistant hepatitis B patients. Gastroenterology 2007;133:1445.

80. Zoulim F, Perrillo R, Hepatitis B. Reflections on the current approach to antiviral therapy. J Hepatol 2008;48(Suppl 1):S2.

81. Fournier C, Zoulim F. Antiviral therapy of chronic hepatitis B: prevention of drug resistance. Clin Liver Dis 2007;11:869.

82. Leigh Brown AJ, Frost SD, Mathews WC, et al. Transmission fitness of drug-resistant human immunodeficiency virus and the prevalence of resistance in the antiretroviral-treated population. J Infect Dis 2003;187:683.

83. Little SJ, Holte S, Routy JP, et al. Antiretroviral-drug resistance among patients recently infected with HIV. N Engl J Med 2002;347:385.

84. Hirsch MS, Brun-Vezinet F, Clotet B, et al. Antiretroviral drug resistance testing in adults infected with human immunodeficiency virus type 1: 2003 recommendations of an International AIDS Society-USA Panel. Clin Infect Dis 2003;37:113.

85. Little SJ, Frost SD, Wong JK, et al. Persistence of transmitted drug resistance among subjects with primary human immunodeficiency virus infection. J Virol 2008;82:5510.

86. Yuen LK, Ayres A, Littlejohn M, et al. SeqHepB: a sequence analysis program and relational database system for chronic hepatitis B. Antiviral Res 2007;75:64.
87. Gauthier J, Bourne EJ, Lutz MW, et al. Quantitation of hepatitis B viremia and emergence of YMDD variants in patients with chronic hepatitis B treated with lamivudine. J Infect Dis 1999;180:1757.
88. Shaw T, Locarnini S. Combination chemotherapy for hepatitis B virus: the path forward? Drugs 2000;60:517.

Chronic Hepatitis B and Hepatocellular Carcinoma

Amy C. McClune, MD*, Myron J. Tong, MD, PhD

KEYWORDS

- Hepatitis B • Hepatitis B carcinogenesis
- Hepatocellular carcinoma

Hepatocellular carcinoma (HCC) is the fifth most common cancer in the world and the third leading cause of cancer-related deaths.[1] More than 80% of HCC cases are from the Asian and African continents, and more than 50% of cases are from mainland China.[2] Approximately 350 million to 400 million persons are chronically infected with hepatitis B virus (HBV), and this virus is the most common cause of HCC worldwide. It is estimated that more than 50% of liver cancers worldwide are attributable to HBV and up to 89% of HBV-related HCC are from developing countries. Recently, increasing trends in HCC incidence have been reported from several Western countries, including France, Australia, and the United States.[3] Factors associated with increased risk for HCC among people with chronic HBV infection include demographic characteristics, host factors, viral-related factors, stage of clinical disease, and lifestyle or environmental influences.

HEPATITIS B VIRUS AND HEPATOCARCINOGENESIS

HBV-associated carcinogenesis is a multifactorial process that involves direct and indirect mechanisms that may act synergistically.[4] Over the last several decades, HBV integration into the host genome, and transactivation of oncogenes by hepatitis B X gene (HBx) protein or by another protein from the pre-S2/S region of the HBV genome, have all been ascribed roles in the pathogenesis of HBV-related HCC.[3] Indirect mechanisms leading to chronic hepatic injury and hepatic regeneration have also been proposed.

The integration of HBV DNA into cellular DNA may be an early event and allows for direct induction of chromosomal translocation, duplication or deletion, and amplification of cellular DNA.[5] These events may also modulate the expression of neighboring cellular genes at sites regulating cell signaling or proliferation. Sequences encoding for

Dumont-UCLA Liver Transplant Center, David Geffen School of Medicine at UCLA, The Pfleger Liver Institute, 200 UCLA Medical Plaza, Suite 214, Los Angeles, CA 90095-7302, USA
* Corresponding author.
E-mail address: amcclune@mednet.ucla.edu

Clin Liver Dis 14 (2010) 461–476
doi:10.1016/j.cld.2010.05.009
1089-3261/10/$ – see front matter © 2010 Elsevier Inc. All rights reserved.

liver.theclinics.com

HBX or pre-S2/S viral proteins are consistently found in a large proportion of tumor cells.[3] The HBx protein is a cytoplasmic protein that may contribute to carcinogenesis through multiple mechanisms, including the modulation of cell signaling pathways, transactivator to a wide range of cellular and viral genes, and inhibitor to DNA repair mechanisms.[4,5]

Cirrhosis is the most important risk factor for HCC. Approximately 90% of HBV-related HCC cases have histologic or clinical evidence of cirrhosis. Necrosis of hepatocytes during chronic infection coupled with rapid regeneration may lead to the accumulation of mutations and selection of clonal tumor expansion with malignant phenotypes.[3] DNA repair may be hindered and the release of reactive oxygen species may also contribute to loss of control of cell growth or apoptosis thereby contributing to tumor development in the cirrhotic liver.[5]

Host Factors

Age
Older age, especially more than 40 years, is strongly associated with an increased incidence of HCC. When compared with the 30 to 39 years age group, several cohort studies have shown that the relative risk for HCC increased from 3.6 to 5.4 in the 40 to 49 years age group and to 8.3 to 17.7 in the 60 years or older age group.[3] However, although less common, HBV-related HCC may still arise during childhood and in patients younger than 40 years of age (**Box 1**).

Gender
Men with chronic HBV infection are at greater risk for developing HCC compared with women. Two Taiwanese studies that followed nearly 4000 subjects with chronic HBV infection for a mean of 11.4 and 12.3 years respectively found that the adjusted relative risk for developing HCC in men was 2.1 (95% CI, 1.3–3.3) and 3.6 (95% CI, 2.4–5.3) compared with women.[3] There are few long-term studies looking at hepatitis B virus and HCC in women. A nationwide, population-based cohort study of more than 1.5 million parous women with chronic hepatitis B in Taiwan conducted for more than 20 years with a mean follow up of 8 years analyzed the association between HCC and hepatitis B surface antigen (HBsAg) status and hepatitis B e antigen (HBeAg) status.[6] In this report, HBsAg positivity was associated with a statistically significant risk for HCC, and this risk was further increased with a positive HBeAg status. Although women who were persistently HBsAg positive had nearly a 3-fold increase in HCC risk compared with those who had HBsAg seroclearance, the loss of hepatitis B surface antigen was still associated with an approximately 8-fold increase risk for HCC when compared with a population who had no evidence for chronic HBV infection. HCC risk was inversely related to parity among Taiwanese mothers, even after accounting for HBsAg status and age.[6]

Race
More than 70% of all newly diagnosed liver cancers occur in Asia, which is also where 75% of the chronically infected HBV population reside.[7] China alone accounts for more than 50% of cases of HCC where the odds ratio for HBV is 12.45 compared with the odds ratio of 4.28 for those with chronic hepatitis C infection.[7] Thus, the primary etiologic agent for HCC in Asia is chronic HBV infection, which is acquired mainly through maternal-fetal transmission. In most Asian countries, HBV usually accounts for 70% to 80% of the HCC cases, with the exception of Japan where chronic HBV infection accounts for only 11% of HCC cases, whereas chronic hepatitis C virus (HCV) accounts for close to 80% of cases.[7]

Box 1
Factors associated with increased risk for hepatocellular carcinoma in patients who are hepatitis B surface antigen positive

1. Host factors
   - Older age
   - Male gender
   - Asian and African ancestry
   - Family history of hepatocellular carcinoma (HCC)
2. Environmental factors
   - Aflatoxin exposure
3. Lifestyle and health-associated factors
   - Alcohol
   - Smoking
   - Diabetes
   - Obesity
4. Clinical factors
   - Cirrhosis
   - Hepatitis C virus (HCV) co-infection
5. Hepatitis B viral factors
   - Hepatitis B e antigen (HBeAg)
   - Hepatitis B virus (HBV) DNA
   - HBV genotype
   - Precore mutation
   - Basal core promoter mutation

In the United States, chronic HBV is the primary etiologic agent in Asian Americans with HCC.[8] In 2006, 13.1% of the population in the Los Angeles area were Asian American and up to 15% of this ethnic group is chronically infected with hepatitis B.[8] Rates of HCC are 2 times higher in Asians than in African Americans and up to 4 times higher than those in Caucasians.[9] In a population of HBV-related HCC cases in a liver cancer clinic in Southern California, 84% of patients were Asian, 10% were Caucasian, and 6% were African American.[10]

Approximately 800 million people live in Africa, which accounts for 12% of the world population. Within this continent, approximately 65 million individuals have chronic hepatitis B infection. The relative risk for an African who is a chronic HBV carrier developing HCC ranges from 9 to 23, with reported age-adjusted rates of HCC in sub-Saharan Africa between 9 and 113 per 100,000 of the population per annum. Perinatal transmission is less common and is only found to be high in infants born to mothers who are hepatitis B e antigen-positive HBV carriers. In African countries, several studies suggest that hepatitis B infection is likely to be acquired by horizontal rather than perinatal transmission. This transmission usually occurs through intrafamilial spread and to a lesser extent by interfamilial routes. Although the exact means of horizontal transmission have not been elucidated, environmental, behavioral, and cultural factors may be involved. Although not substantiated, risk behaviors that may be associated with HBV infection include sharing of bath towels, chewing gum, partially eating sweets, dental cleaning material, and biting fingernails in conjunction with scratching the backs of HBV carriers. Cultural practices, such as scarification, tattooing, and use of sharp objects, increase the risk for HBV infection. Iatrogenic procedures, including tonsillectomy, indiscriminate injections, or the reuse of nonsterilized syringes, have also increased the risk for HBV transmission.[11]

Family history of hepatocellular carcinoma

Several studies have reported an increased risk for HCC in first-degree relatives of subjects with HBV-related HCC. A large case-control study in Taiwan looked at data from first-degree relatives of 553 HBV carriers with HCC and 4686 HBV carriers without HCC who served as controls. First-degree relatives of case subjects were more likely to have HCC. This finding was particularly notable in siblings, although it was also observed in parents. Certain transmissible genetic factors therefore may be associated with the development of HCC in some families of HBV carriers with a family history of HCC.[12] Another case-control study in the United States observed a relationship between chronic HBV/HCV infection and subjects' family history of liver cancer, which was independent of each other's effects, thereby implying that individuals with both of these risk factors are at the highest risk for developing HCC, especially at a young age.[13] This synergism was also seen in an Italian cohort by Donato and colleagues[14] who reported an odds ratio of 70.1 among Italian individuals who had HBV infection and a family history of HCC.

Lifestyle and environmental factors

Alcohol consumption is common in the United States and Western Europe and its use has been increasing in Asia over the last 30 years, most notably in men.[15] Chronic alcohol use in excess of 80 g/d for longer than 10 years increases the risk for developing HCC approximately 5-fold.[15] A population-based cohort study from Korea revealed an increasing risk for HCC in HBV carriers who drank 50 g/d or more of alcohol. A longitudinal study from Japan in the 1970s compared 341 hepatitis B surface antigen-positive blood donors who consumed more than 27 g/d of alcohol to a group of abstinent hepatitis B subjects and found a 5-fold increase in the relative risk for developing HCC in the former group.[15] In a case control study, Hassan and colleagues[16] reported a synergistic relationship between chronic hepatitis viral infection (both hepatitis B and C) and chronic alcohol consumption for the risk for HCC development.

Smoking

Although the data is conflicting, tobacco use may also increase the risk for HCC in patients with chronic hepatitis B. In a study of 12,000 Taiwanese men, there was a 1.5-fold increased risk for HCC among cigarette smokers compared with nonsmokers.[17] However, a population-based cohort study of more than 3500 Taiwanese men who were HBsAg carriers revealed that smoking did not affect the risk for HCC after adjustment for other known HCC risk factors.[18]

Aflatoxins

Aflatoxins are known to be potent hepatocarcinogens in animals, and human exposure to these mycotoxins may occur through ingestion of moldy foods resulting from humid storage of various grains, especially in sub-Sahara Africa and Southeast Asia. A large prospective cohort study in Shanghai using a urinary biomarker of exposure was one of the first studies linking dietary aflatoxin exposure to HCC development in individuals with chronic HBV infection.[19] Another report revealed that even modest levels of aflatoxin exposure may increase HCC risk in men infected with HBV up to 3-fold.[20]

Diabetes and Obesity

Other conditions aside from viral hepatitis and alcohol may predispose to HCC. Diabetes is part of the metabolic syndrome and has been identified as a potential risk factor for HCC. In a large population study examining the association between diabetes and HCC in the United States, Davila and colleagues found that diabetes is an independent risk factor for HCC, regardless of the presence of HCV, HBV, alcoholic liver disease, or cirrhosis.[16,21] Furthermore, Hassan and colleagues[16] reported synergy between heavy alcohol consumption, chronic viral hepatitis, and diabetes in the etiology of HCC, and this was independent of each other's effect. A meta-analysis by El-Serag and colleagues reviewing epidemiologic studies looking at the association of diabetes and HCC revealed that diabetes is associated with an approximately 2.5-fold increase in the risk for HCC.[22] However, it is difficult in these case-control studies to examine not only the temporal relationship between an exposure, such as diabetes, and an outcome, such as HCC, but to also account for confounding factors, such as diet, exercise and obesity. Increasingly, components of the metabolic syndrome, such as insulin resistance, hypertension, obesity, and dyslipidemia, are being linked to a variety of cancers. A large prospective cohort study of more than 900,000 participants over a 16-year follow-up in the Cancer Prevention Study II found significantly higher rates of death for all cancers, and the mortality rate from HCC showed a 5-fold increase among men and women with a body mass index (BMI) of 35 to 40 compared with those having a normal BMI.[23] As viral-related cases of HCC decrease, there may be increasing evidence for obesity-related HCC in the future.

Viral Factors

In a landmark prospective study published in 1981, Beasley and colleagues[24] reported on 22,707 Chinese men in Taiwan of whom 3454 were HBsAg-positive and showed that the incidence of HCC was profoundly higher in this population compared with non-HBV carriers. Subsequent epidemiologic studies have confirmed that HBsAg positivity is one of the most important risk factors for HCC. The presence of HBeAg in serum indicates active viral replication in hepatocytes and therefore is a surrogate marker for HBV DNA. A prospective study of close to 12,000 Taiwanese men followed for approximately 10 year revealed that HBeAg positivity was associated with an increased risk for HCC.[17] Although not directly tested, this report suggested that the younger the age of HBeAg seroconversion to anti-HBeAg, the lower the risk for HCC. The effect of HBeAg status remained an independent predictor after adjusting for important covariates, including HCV status, alcohol intake, and cigarette smoking.

The Risk Evaluation of Viral Load Elevation and Associated Liver Disease/Cancer-Hepatitis B (REVEAL-HBV) study followed 4155 HBsAg-seropositive adults aged 30 to 64 years from 1991 until 2004. The incidence of progression to cirrhosis and development of HCC were the two major outcomes in the REVEAL-HBV study. The investigators noted that increasing the HBV DNA level was one of the strongest independent predictors related to progression to cirrhosis.[25] Also, the HBV DNA level remained an independent predictor of HCC even after adjusting for known covariates, including sex, age, cigarette smoking, alcohol consumption, HBeAg status, serum alanine aminotransferase level, and the presence of cirrhosis at baseline. In this cohort of subjects, it was concluded that an HBV DNA level greater than 10,000 copies/mL was associated with a significantly increased risk for progression to cirrhosis and for development of HCC.[18]

Other viral factors may predispose certain chronic hepatitis B carriers toward development of HCC. A dual mutation in the basal core promoter (BCP) region of the HBV genome involving an A-T substitution at nucleotide 1762 and a G-A substitution at nucleotide 1764 may be one of these factors. Also, a mutation in the precore (PC) region of the HBV genome involving a G-A substitution at nucleotide 1896 has been described in patients with HBeAg-negative chronic hepatitis. In a study looking at potential viral factors that might predispose to HCC in a predominantly Asian group, 67 chronic carriers previously followed for a mean of 112 months were compared with 101 subjects who were HBsAg-positive with HCC. Higher frequencies of PC A1896 mutants, BCP T1762/A1764 mutants, the presence of genotype C, and higher levels of HBV DNA were detected more often in subjects with HCC compared with chronic carriers.[26]

Six genotypes (A through F) of hepatitis B have been identified. However, their role in influencing clinical outcomes in patients with chronic HBV infection is still under investigation. Specific HBV genotypes may predispose individuals to more severe liver disease or to the development of HCC. A Taiwanese cross-sectional study revealed that there was strong association of genotype B with the earlier development of HCC in younger subjects (<50 years of age) and in subjects who were not cirrhotic. Genotype C was more prevalent in subjects with cirrhosis, suggesting an association with more severe liver disease and subsequent development of HCC. Although additional population-based prospective longitudinal studies are needed, these findings indicate possible pathogenetic differences among HBV genotypes.[27]

Lastly, with respect to viral factors, a small proportion of subjects often estimated between 0.1% and 1.2% in Asian countries with chronic hepatitis B infection may experience HBsAg seroclearance. The outcomes after HBsAg seroclearance are generally favorable. In the United States, 35 subjects with a history of chronic hepatitis B who were followed between 1976 and 2008 at a community liver clinic subsequently lost HBsAg, had negative viral DNA levels, and were anti-HBeAg positive. Four subjects with cirrhosis subsequently developed HCC despite HBsAg seroclearance. Therefore, continued surveillance for HCC is important especially if cirrhosis is already present at the time of HBsAg loss.[28]

SURVEILLANCE

The objective of surveillance for HCC is to reduce mortality in patients who have the potential for developing this malignancy. Prospective studies have shown that the annual rate for HCC development in patients with HBsAg-positive cirrhosis is up to 4% per year.[29] In a recent United States report, the rate of HCC development in a population of untreated subjects with HBV cirrhosis was 4.4% per year.[30] Serum alpha fetoprotein (AFP) testing and abdominal ultrasound examination are the two most commonly used modalities for HCC surveillance. A large randomized trial in Shanghai demonstrated that routine imaging with abdominal ultrasound and serum AFP every 6 months significantly improved survival, and the HCC mortality rate was reduced by 37%.[31] Therefore, patients who are HBsAg positive who are at high risk for HCC development should undergo routine surveillance for HCC (**Box 2**).

Serum AFP has been a commonly used serum marker for HCC detection since 1960. However, AFP may not be elevated in up to 30% of patients with HCC. The AFP test for HCC has a sensitivity of 39% to 65% and a specificity of 76% to 94% in previously published studies. Recently, the American Association for the Study of Liver Diseases (AASLD) and European Association for the Study of the Liver (EASL) guidelines recommended against using AFP alone for HCC surveillance. However,

---

Box 2
Surveillance for HCC in patients with HBsAg

1. Surveillance every 3 to 6 months
   - Patients with cirrhosis
   - All HBsAg positive
   - After HBsAg seroclearance
2. Surveillance every 6 months
   - Patients with chronic hepatitis B
   - Men aged 40 years or older
   - Women aged 50 years or older
   - Family history of HCC
3. Surveillance every 12 months
   - Patients with HBsAg + immune tolerance
   - HBsAg + inactive carriers

---

levels of AFP greater than 400 ng/mL should be highly suspicious for HCC, and further imaging studies with CT scan or MRI should be performed immediately.

In a prospective surveillance study between 1991 and 1998, 602 subjects with chronic viral hepatitis were enrolled and the mean follow-up time was 34.5 ± 24 months.[32] In this report, 31 subjects developed HCC, however, only 4 of these subjects had AFP levels greater than 400 ng/mL, which is considered diagnostic for HCC. Eighteen subjects had values between 8 and 400 ng/mL and 7 subjects had normal levels below 8 ng/mL. The positive predictive value of AFP for HCC detection was low and therefore the measurement of AFP alone is not a good test for detecting early HCC. During the surveillance period, the positive predictive value of ultrasound (US) was 78% with a sensitivity of 100% and a specificity of 98%. Only 9 false-positive US tests out of a total of 1388 US examinations (0.6%) were observed in contrast to a high number of false-positive AFP tests that were found during this study. In an Asian American HBV population in the United States, surveillance for HCC with both AFP and ultrasound examination identified subjects with smaller tumor burdens who were able to receive therapies, which significantly improved survival.[8] In this report, significant survival benefits were noted in those subjects whose HCC was detected by surveillance, in subjects with a Child-Turcotte-Pugh class A, and in those whose tumors were within the Milan and University of California, San Francisco (UCSF) criteria (**Fig. 1**).

DIAGNOSIS

Given the poor performance of AFP to detect HCC, other serum markers have been proposed although their clinical utility has not been fully elucidated (see **Box 1**). AFP-L3 and des-γ-carboxyprothrombin (DCP) are 2 tumor markers that have received considerable attention recently although there have been conflicting results. One study found that DCP had the highest sensitivity and positive predictive value for diagnosing HCC when compared with AFP and AFP-L3.[33] This study also revealed that DCP directly correlated with tumor size. However, a nested case control study within the Hepatitis C Antiviral Long-term Treatment Against Cirrhosis (HALT-C) trial concluded that DCP was not superior to AFP in detecting early HCC among subjects

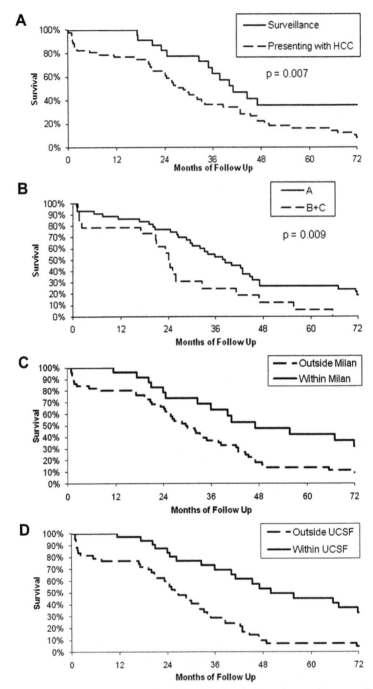

Fig. 1. (*A*) Survival of patients who presented with HCC to those detected by surveillance. (*B*) Survival of patients with HCC by Child-Turcotte-Pugh class. (*C*) Survival of patients with HCC by Milan criteria. (*D*) Survival of patients with HCC by University of California San Francisco criteria.

with advanced hepatitis C.[34] However, consideration was given to DCP, and AFP may be complementary but further prospective studies are needed to determine whether combining both markers improves early detection of HCC.

The diagnosis of HCC is initially confirmed by radiologic imaging. Common imaging modalities employed for HCC diagnosis include US, triple phase CT, and dynamic MRI. A recent prospective study showed that MRI had a sensitivity of 75% and a specificity of 76% for diagnosis of HCC compared with triple phase CT, which had a sensitivity of 61% and specificity of 66%.[35] Other studies have also confirmed that MRI may be slightly better than CT at diagnosing HCC.[36,37] Arterial enhancement with washout of a mass in a patient who is cirrhotic has a sensitivity of approximately 80% and a specificity of nearly 95% to 100% for HCC.[38] If a lesion does not meet this criteria and the AFP is not markedly elevated, then the lesion should undergo biopsy examination. The accuracy of MRI and CT for diagnosis of HCC is affected by the size of the liver mass. MRI has been reported to have a detection rate for HCC of greater than 95% in tumors larger than 2 cm; however, this rate is reduced to 33% if tumors are less than 2 cm.[39]

Hepatic lesions ranging from 1 to 2 cm in size may be considered diagnostic of HCC if the characteristic arterial enhancement pattern is seen on 2 different imaging modalities (ie, CT scan and MRI). A biopsy may be considered if only 1 of the imaging studies illustrates this vascular pattern. Hepatic lesions less than 1 cm in size need to be followed up every 3 months to determine if interval growth is suggestive of malignancy. If a lesion demonstrates stability after 2 years of follow-up, then the return to standard surveillance protocol every 6 to 12 months is recommended.[39] A diagnosis of HCC can be made in patients who have a hepatic mass greater than 2 cm that is identified on 1 dynamic imaging study demonstrating a typical vascular pattern with arterial enhancement followed by venous phase washout. If an atypical vascular pattern is visualized, a biopsy would be recommended.

Fine needle aspiration biopsy and standard liver biopsy allow for cytologic examination of a suspected lesion. However, diagnostic efficacy ranges from 60% to 90% and is dependent on the size of the lesion, the diameter of the needle, and the skill of the operator. Complications associated with liver biopsy are low with mortality estimated below 1% and the risk for tumor seeding along the needle tract has been estimated up to 3%. Microscopically, HCC cells have an elevated nuclear-to-cytoplasmic ratio, trabecular architecture, atypical naked nuclei, and peripheral wrapping.[40]

TREATMENT

Treatment of HCC needs to be individualized based on the underlying liver disease, tumor characteristics, overall side effects, and patient performance status (**Box 3**). Therapeutic goals of various modalities differ and range from palliative to curative and from targeted to systemic in scope. The management of HCC is multidisciplinary and should include hepatologists, surgeons, oncologists, pathologists, and interventional radiologists. A University of California, Los Angeles (UCLA) algorithm for treatment of HCC has recently been described (**Fig. 2**).[41]

Hepatic Resection

Selection of patients is a critical component to the success of hepatic resection of HCC. Resection is the treatment of choice for patients with HCC who do not have cirrhosis because of the fact that the residual liver has well-preserved function. However, this group of patients accounts for only 5% of patients in Western countries and 40% of patients in Asian countries.[42] Patients with cirrhosis are at risk for hepatic decompensation after surgical resection given the poor regenerative capability of the residual cirrhotic liver. Consequently, selection criteria for patients with cirrhosis are often employed and include a normal bilirubin value and the absence of portal hypertension. The latter is often inferred by a platelet count greater than $100,000/mm^3$ and the absence of esophageal varices, or if a direct measurement of the hepatic vein pressure gradient of less than 10 mmHg can be obtained.[38] This select group of patients may achieve overall survival rates higher than 70% at 5 years.[43] The risk for tumor recurrence is related to many variables, including tumor size, tumor number, width of tumor-free resection margin, and the presence of macrovascular or microvascular

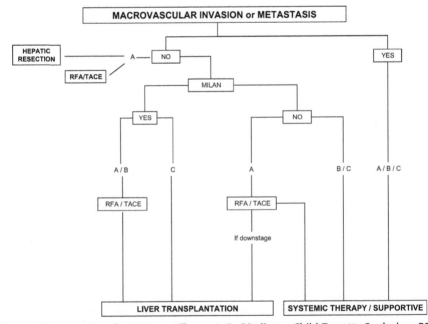

Fig. 2. UCLA algorithm for HCC surveillance. A, B, C indicates Child-Turcotte-Pugh class; RFA, radiofrequency ablation; TACE, transcatheter arterial chemoembolization.

invasion.[44] HCC recurrence rates of 50% at 3 years and 70% at 5 years have been reported after resection.[44,45] Currently, there is interest in developing adjuvant or molecular targeted therapies in an attempt to prevent HCC recurrence after resection.

Liver Transplantation

Liver transplantation offers the optimal treatment for HCC because it is curative and also eliminates the underlying cirrhosis. The landmark study by Mazzaferro and colleagues in 1996 showed that when liver transplantation was performed for a single HCC less than or equal to 5 cm, or up to 3 lesions, each less than 3 cm in size, survival rates were greater than 70% at 4 years and recurrence was less than 15%.[46] This criteria, known as the Milan criteria, has been accepted by the United Network for Organ Sharing (UNOS) for the selection of patients with HCC for orthotopic liver transplantation (OLT). Patients who meet the Milan criteria are eligible to receive a Model for End-Stage Liver Disease (MELD) score of 22, which is equivalent to a 15% probability of death within 3 months. Therefore, the MELD score for patients remaining on the wait list is then increased 10% every 3 months to reflect the increase in the pretransplant mortality risk.

Yao and colleagues[47] at UCSF proposed an expansion of the Milan criteria to a single tumor less than or equal to 6.5 cm or up to 3 tumors, the largest less than or equal to 4.5 cm, with a total tumor diameter of less than 8 cm.[47] Reported long-term survival posttransplant is similar to patients meeting the Milan criteria. These criteria were originally derived from tumor characteristics based on explant data and subsequently validated by a UCSF cohort with selection criteria based on preoperative imaging studies. Similarly, a large series from UCLA looked at all subjects (N = 467) undergoing OLT for HCC over a 22-year period and outcomes were compared for subjects who either met Milan criteria, UCSF criteria, or actually exceeded UCSF criteria.[48] Subjects meeting Milan criteria had similar 5-year posttransplant survival compared with subjects meeting UCSF criteria by explant pathology and preoperative imaging. Survival was less than 50% at 5 years for subjects with HCC beyond UCSF criteria. Further studies will be helpful before expansion of the current criteria for liver transplantation.

Downstaging of tumor size by using locoregional modalities to meet Milan criteria appears to be an encouraging option for patients subsequently undergoing OLT. It is estimated that approximately 70% of patients may be successfully downstaged by using radiofrequency ablation (RFA), percutaneous ethanol injection (PEI), or transcatheter arterial chemoembolization (TACE). Initial tumor free and overall survival outcomes have been similar when compared with patients transplanted within Milan criteria.[47] However, longer follow-up will be required to assess the risk for HCC recurrence before downstaging can be recommended and included in current guidelines.

Locoregional Therapies

Various locoregional therapies have been used to treat HCC, including cryoablation, microwave ablation, radiotherapy, PEI, yttrium-90 microspheres, RFA, and TACE. The most commonly used percutaneous methods to induce tumor necrosis are PEI and RFA. PEI is usually performed under ultrasound guidance and consists of injecting ethanol directly into the lesion. It is reported to achieve coagulative necrosis in almost 100% of tumors less than 2 cm and 70% to 80% of tumors 3 cm or less in size. Its efficacy drops to 50% in tumors between 3 to 5 cm.[49–51] The procedure is usually well tolerated and has few side effects. However, repeated injections are often required and the best survival for this technique is mostly limited to less than 3 tumors, each of which is less than 3 cm in size.[52]

RFA has emerged as a treatment of choice when compared with PEI. RFA achieves the same efficacy as PEI with tumors less than 2 cm while requiring a fewer number of sessions and it is also more effective in ablating larger tumors.[53] There have been several recent randomized trials, mostly in Asia, comparing RFA and PEI treatments in subjects with HCC less than 4 cm. A superior survival benefit was seen with RFA compared with PEI, with 4-year survival of 74% achieved with RFA.[53,54] RFA was also superior in lower tumor recurrence. In patients treated with RFA, local recurrence rates have reportedly ranged from 8% to 14% at 2 to 3 years compared with rates of 22% to 34% in patients treated with PEI.[38]

Two randomized controlled trials compared RFA with surgical resection for tumors less than or equal to 2 cm and both studies found no significant differences in overall survival or recurrence-free survival.[55,56] Lower hospitalization rates and fewer complication rates were also seen in subjects treated with RFA. In addition, RFA may have a role in patients awaiting liver transplantation. Given the limited supply of donor organs and subsequently prolonged waiting times for liver transplant, high drop-out rates often occur because of tumor progression. A study at UCLA examined the outcome of 87 tumors treated with RFA in 52 liver transplant candidates and complete tumor coagulation was observed in 85% of subjects based on postablation imaging.[57] After a mean of 12.7 months on the waiting list, only 3 of 52 subjects dropped out because of tumor progression. Forty-one subjects subsequently underwent liver transplant with 1- year and 3-year survival rates of 85% and 76% respectively, without any recurrence of HCC. Although more studies are indicated, RFA may serve as either a therapeutic option for patients with small tumors who are not optimal surgical candidates or as bridging therapy for unresectable HCC in patients within Milan criteria who are awaiting liver transplantation.

Transarterial embolization or chemoembolization is considered a safe and effective therapeutic option in patients with preserved liver function and in patients who do not have evidence of vascular invasion, cancer-related symptoms, or extrahepatic spread of HCC.[58] The concept of embolization is to induce ischemic tumor necrosis by acute arterial occlusion. This procedure may be performed alone or in combination with a selective intra-arterial chemotherapy agent, such as doxorubicin, cisplatin, or mitomycin, and a contrast agent, such as Lipiodol. TACE may provide palliative benefits for patients with intermediate-stage HCC who are not eligible for OLT. It can also be performed in patients with early stage HCC who are not candidates for RFA because of tumor proximity to the gallbladder, biliary tree, diaphragm, or a blood vessel. TACE is also used for downstaging of tumors that exceed criteria for liver transplant although specific treatment recommendations in this area are still considered investigational.

In one of the largest prospective cohort studies enrolling 8510 subjects who received TACE for unresectable HCC, the median survival was found to be 34 months with a 5-year survival of 26%.[59] Currently there is little data to guide the selection of a specific chemotherapeutic agent; however, benefit has been demonstrated in at least 2 randomized trials as compared with the use of embolization alone.[60,61] Reported adverse effects from TACE occur in approximately 10% of treated patients and include nausea, vomiting, bone marrow depression, alopecia, and ischemic cholecystitis.[62] More than 50% of patients treated with TACE experience a postembolization syndrome that includes fever, abdominal pain, and ileus. Overall treatment-related mortality has been estimated at less than 5%.

Systemic Therapy

Advanced HCC or progression of HCC after locoregional therapy has a poor prognosis. Various chemotherapeutic and hormonal agents have been investigated as systemic therapy for HCC in several randomized controlled trials. Agents, such as doxorubicin, tamoxifen, and fluorouracil, have essentially shown low response rates and no survival benefit in treating HCC compared with appropriate controls.

Molecular-targeted therapies that interrupt pathways critical to cancer progression are being developed and provide hope for improved outcomes. The molecular pathogenesis of HCC has illuminated the importance of growth-receptor signaling and the inactivation of tumor suppressor genes. The most promising agent, sorafenib, is an oral multikinase inhibitor that inhibits tumor cell proliferation and angiogenesis. In the multicenter, Sorafenib Hepatocellular Carcinoma Assessment Randomized Protocol (SHARP) study, sorafenib was studied in a randomized controlled trial of 602 subjects with advanced HCC and demonstrated a 3-month survival improvement compared with placebo.[63] The Asia-Pacific study was performed at 23 sites and was designed in parallel with the SHARP study to assess the efficacy and safety of sorafenib in subjects with advanced HCC from a different geographic region.[64] Similar to the SHARP trial, sorafenib significantly prolonged overall survival compared with placebo and was generally well tolerated. Other agents in phase II studies include anti-epidermal growth factor receptor agents, such as erlotinib and gefitinib; antiangiogenic agents, such as bevacizumab and sunitinib; and mTOR inhibitors, such as everolimus and termsiroloimus.[63] Sorafenib is the first systemic therapy to prolong survival in patients with advanced HCC, thereby representing a breakthrough in the treatment of this complex disease. Given that the number of HCC patients will continue to increase over the next decade, more studies evaluating the efficacy of different molecular targets alone or in combination with either surgical or locoregional therapies will be required.

REFERENCES

1. Parkin DM. Global cancer statistics in the year 2000. Lancet Oncol 2001;2(9): 533–43.
2. El-Serag HB. Epidemiology of hepatocellular carcinoma in USA. Hepatol Res 2007;37(Suppl 2):S88–94.
3. Nguyen VT, Law MG, Dore GJ. Hepatitis B-related hepatocellular carcinoma: epidemiological characteristics and disease burden. J Viral Hepat 2009;16(7): 453–63.
4. Lupberger J, Hildt E. Hepatitis B virus-induced oncogenesis. World J Gastroenterol 2007;13(1):74–81.
5. Chan HL, Sung JJ. Hepatocellular carcinoma and hepatitis B virus. Semin Liver Dis 2006;26(2):153–61.
6. Fwu CW, Chien YC, Kirk GD, et al. Hepatitis B virus infection and hepatocellular carcinoma among parous Taiwanese women: nationwide cohort study. J Natl Cancer Inst 2009;101(14):1019–27.
7. Yuen MF, Hou JL, Chutaputti A. Hepatocellular carcinoma in the Asia pacific region. J Gastroenterol Hepatol 2009;24(3):346–53.
8. Tong MJ, Sun HE, Hsien C, et al. Surveillance for hepatocellular carcinoma improves survival in Asian-American patients with hepatitis B: results from a community-based clinic. Dig Dis Sci 2010;55(3):826–35.
9. El-Serag HB. Hepatocellular carcinoma: recent trends in the United States. Gastroenterology 2004;127(5 Suppl 1):S27–34.
10. Barazani Y, Hiatt JR, Tong MJ, et al. Chronic viral hepatitis and hepatocellular carcinoma. World J Surg 2007;31(6):1243–8.

11. Kramvis A, Kew MC. Epidemiology of hepatitis B virus in Africa, its genotypes and clinical associations of genotypes. Hepatol Res 2007;37(S1):S9–19.

12. Yu MW, Chang HC, Liaw YF, et al. Familial risk of hepatocellular carcinoma among chronic hepatitis B carriers and their relatives. J Natl Cancer Inst 2000;92(14): 1159–64.

13. Hassan MM, Spitz MR, Thomas MB, et al. The association of family history of liver cancer with hepatocellular carcinoma: a case-control study in the United States. J Hepatol 2009;50(2):334–41.

14. Donato F, Gelatti U, Chiesa R, et al. A case-control study on family history of liver cancer as a risk factor for hepatocellular carcinoma in North Italy. Brescia HCC Study. Cancer Causes Control 1999;10(5):417–21.

15. Morgan TR, Mandayam S, Jamal MM. Alcohol and hepatocellular carcinoma. Gastroenterology 2004;127(5 Suppl 1):S87–96.

16. Hassan MM, Hwang LY, Hatten CJ, et al. Risk factors for hepatocellular carcinoma: synergism of alcohol with viral hepatitis and diabetes mellitus. Hepatology 2002;36(5):1206–13.

17. Yang HI, Lu SN, Liaw YF, et al. Hepatitis B e antigen and the risk of hepatocellular carcinoma. N Engl J Med 2002;347(3):168–74.

18. Chen CJ, Yang HI, Su J, et al. Risk of hepatocellular carcinoma across a biological gradient of serum hepatitis B virus DNA level. JAMA 2006;295(1):65–73.

19. Yu MC, Yuan JM. Environmental factors and risk for hepatocellular carcinoma. Gastroenterology 2004;127(5 Suppl 1):S72–78.

20. Fattovich G, Bortolotti F, Donato F. Natural history of chronic hepatitis B: special emphasis on disease progression and prognostic factors. J Hepatol 2008; 48(2):335–52.

21. Davila JA, Morgan RO, Shaib Y, et al. Diabetes increases the risk of hepatocellular carcinoma in the United States: a population based case control study. Gut 2005;54(4):533–9.

22. El-Serag HB, Hampel H, Javadi F. The association between diabetes and hepatocellular carcinoma: a systematic review of epidemiologic evidence. Clin Gastroenterol Hepatol 2006;4(3):369–80.

23. Calle EE, Rodriguez C, Walker-Thurmond K, et al. Overweight, obesity, and mortality from cancer in a prospectively studied cohort of U.S. adults. N Engl J Med 2003;348(17):1625–38.

24. Beasley RP, Hwang LY, Lin CC, et al. Hepatocellular carcinoma and hepatitis B virus. A prospective study of 22 707 men in Taiwan. Lancet 1981;2(8256): 1129–33.

25. Iloeje UH, Yang HI, Su J, et al. Predicting cirrhosis risk based on the level of circulating hepatitis B viral load. Gastroenterology 2006;130(3):678–86.

26. Tong MJ, Blatt LM, Kao JH, et al. Basal core promoter T1762/A1764 and precore A1896 gene mutations in hepatitis B surface antigen-positive hepatocellular carcinoma: a comparison with chronic carriers. Liver Int 2007;27(10): 1356–63.

27. Kao JH, Chen PJ, Lai MY, et al. Hepatitis B genotypes correlate with clinical outcomes in patients with chronic hepatitis B. Gastroenterology 2000;118(3): 554–9.

28. Tong MJ, Nguyen MO, Tong LT, et al. Development of hepatocellular carcinoma after seroclearance of hepatitis B surface antigen. Clin Gastroenterol Hepatol 2009;7(8):889–93.

29. Marrero JA, Welling T. Modern diagnosis and management of hepatocellular carcinoma. Clin Liver Dis 2009;13(2):233–47.

30. Tong MJ, Hsien C, Song JJ, et al. Factors associated with progression to hepatocellular carcinoma and to death from liver complications in patients with HBsAg-positive cirrhosis. Dig Dis Sci 2009;54(6):1337–46.
31. Zhang BH, Yang BH, Tang ZY. Randomized controlled trial of screening for hepatocellular carcinoma. J Cancer Res Clin Oncol 2004;130(7):417–22.
32. Tong MJ, Blatt LM, Kao VW. Surveillance for hepatocellular carcinoma in patients with chronic viral hepatitis in the United States of America. J Gastroenterol Hepatol 2001;16(5):553–9.
33. Durazo FA, Blatt LM, Corey WG, et al. Des-gamma-carboxyprothrombin, alphafetoprotein and AFP-L3 in patients with chronic hepatitis, cirrhosis and hepatocellular carcinoma. J Gastroenterol Hepatol 2008;23(10):1541–8.
34. Lok AS, Sterling RK, Everhart JE, et al. Des-gamma-carboxy prothrombin and alpha-fetoprotein as biomarkers for the early detection of hepatocellular carcinoma. Gastroenterology 2010;138(2):493–502.
35. Burrel M, Llovet JM, Ayuso C, et al. MRI angiography is superior to helical CT for detection of HCC prior to liver transplantation: an explant correlation. Hepatology 2003;38(4):1034–42.
36. Rode A, Bancel B, Douek P, et al. Small nodule detection in cirrhotic livers: evaluation with US, spiral CT, and MRI and correlation with pathologic examination of explanted liver. J Comput Assist Tomogr 2001;25(3):327–36.
37. Krinsky GA, Lee VS, Theise ND, et al. Hepatocellular carcinoma and dysplastic nodules in patients with cirrhosis: prospective diagnosis with MR imaging and explantation correlation. Radiology 2001;219(2):445–54.
38. El-Serag HB, Marrero JA, Rudolph L, et al. Diagnosis and treatment of hepatocellular carcinoma. Gastroenterology 2008;134(6):1752–63.
39. Bruix J, Sherman M. Management of hepatocellular carcinoma. Hepatology 2005; 42(5):1208–36.
40. Gomaa AI, Khan SA, Leen EL, et al. Diagnosis of hepatocellular carcinoma. World J Gastroenterol 2009;15(11):1301–14.
41. Tong MJ, Chavalitdhamrong D, Lu DS, et al. Survival in Asian Americans after treatments for hepatocellular carcinoma: a seven-year experience at UCLA. J Clin Gastroenterol 2010;44(3):e63–70.
42. Bolondi L, Sofia S, Siringo S, et al. Surveillance programme of cirrhotic patients for early diagnosis and treatment of hepatocellular carcinoma: a cost effectiveness analysis. Gut 2001;48(2):251–9.
43. Llovet JM, Bru C, Bruix J. Prognosis of hepatocellular carcinoma: the BCLC staging classification. Semin Liver Dis 1999;19(3):329–38.
44. Mendizabal M, Reddy KR. Current management of hepatocellular carcinoma. Med Clin North Am 2009;93(4):885–900, viii.
45. Bruix J, Sherman M, Llovet JM, et al. Clinical management of hepatocellular carcinoma. Conclusions of the Barcelona-2000 EASL conference. European Association for the Study of the Liver. J Hepatol 2001;35(3):421–30.
46. Mazzaferro V, Regalia E, Doci R, et al. Liver transplantation for the treatment of small hepatocellular carcinomas in patients with cirrhosis. N Engl J Med 1996; 334(11):693–9.
47. Yao FY, Ferrell L, Bass NM, et al. Liver transplantation for hepatocellular carcinoma: expansion of the tumor size limits does not adversely impact survival. Hepatology 2001;33(6):1394–403.
48. Duffy JP, Vardanian A, Benjamin E, et al. Liver transplantation criteria for hepatocellular carcinoma should be expanded: a 22-year experience with 467 patients at UCLA. Ann Surg 2007;246(3):502–9 [discussion: 509–11].

49. Ishii H, Okada S, Nose H, et al. Local recurrence of hepatocellular carcinoma after percutaneous ethanol injection. Cancer 1996;77(9):1792–6.
50. Livraghi T, Bolondi L, Lazzaroni S, et al. Percutaneous ethanol injection in the treatment of hepatocellular carcinoma in cirrhosis. A study on 207 patients. Cancer 1992;69(4):925–9.
51. Vilana R, Bruix J, Bru C, et al. Tumor size determines the efficacy of percutaneous ethanol injection for the treatment of small hepatocellular carcinoma. Hepatology 1992;16(2):353–7.
52. Ryu M, Shimamura Y, Kinoshita T, et al. Therapeutic results of resection, transcatheter arterial embolization and percutaneous transhepatic ethanol injection in 3225 patients with hepatocellular carcinoma: a retrospective multicenter study. Jpn J Clin Oncol 1997;27(4):251–7.
53. Lin SM, Lin CJ, Lin CC, et-al. Radiofrequency ablation improves prognosis compared with ethanol injection for hepatocellular carcinoma < or =4 cm. Gastroenterology 2004;127(6):1714–23.
54. Shiina S, Teratani T, Obi S, et al. A randomized controlled trial of radiofrequency ablation with ethanol injection for small hepatocellular carcinoma. Gastroenterology 2005;129(1):122–30.
55. Chen MS, Li JQ, Zheng Y, et al. A prospective randomized trial comparing percutaneous local ablative therapy and partial hepatectomy for small hepatocellular carcinoma. Ann Surg 2006;243(3):321–8.
56. Livraghi T, Meloni F, Di Stasi M, et al. Sustained complete response and complications rates after radiofrequency ablation of very early hepatocellular carcinoma in cirrhosis: is resection still the treatment of choice? Hepatology 2008;47(1):82–9.
57. Lu DS, Yu NC, Raman SS, et al. Percutaneous radiofrequency ablation of hepatocellular carcinoma as a bridge to liver transplantation. Hepatology 2005;41(5):1130–7.
58. Llovet JM, Bruix J. Systematic review of randomized trials for unresectable hepatocellular carcinoma: chemoembolization improves survival. Hepatology 2003;37(2):429–42.
59. Takayasu K, Arii S, Ikai I, et al. Prospective cohort study of transarterial chemoembolization for unresectable hepatocellular carcinoma in 8510 patients. Gastroenterology 2006;131(2):461–9.
60. Lo CM, Ngan H, Tso WK, et al. Randomized controlled trial of transarterial lipiodol chemoembolization for unresectable hepatocellular carcinoma. Hepatology 2002;35(5):1164–71.
61. Llovet JM, Real MI, Montana X, et al. Arterial embolisation or chemoembolisation versus symptomatic treatment in patients with unresectable hepatocellular carcinoma: a randomised controlled trial. Lancet 2002;359(9319):1734–9.
62. Molinari M, Kachura JR, Dixon E, et al. Transarterial chemoembolisation for advanced hepatocellular carcinoma: results from a North American cancer centre. Clin Oncol (R Coll Radiol) 2006;18(9):684–92.
63. Llovet JM, Ricci S, Mazzaferro V, et al. Sorafenib in advanced hepatocellular carcinoma. N Engl J Med 2008;359(4):378–90.
64. Cheng AL, Kang YK, Chen Z, et al. Efficacy and safety of sorafenib in patients in the Asia-Pacific region with advanced hepatocellular carcinoma: a phase III randomised, double-blind, placebo-controlled trial. Lancet Oncol 2009;10(1):25–34.

Management of End-Stage Liver Disease in Chronic Hepatitis B

Hui-Hui Tan, MBBS, MRCP[a],*, Paul Martin, MD, FRCP, FRCPI[b]

KEYWORDS

- Hepatitis B • Liver transplantation • End-stage liver disease
- Cirrhosis • Antiviral therapy

Chronic hepatitis B virus (HBV) is the most common cause of chronic viral hepatitis and end-stage liver disease worldwide, with more than 350 million individuals chronically infected.[1,2] For details on the disease burden of HBV infection in the United States, see the article by Kim elsewhere in this issue. Chronic HBV may result in cirrhosis, liver failure, or hepatocellular carcinoma (HCC).[3] Hepatic decompensation usually presents 3 to 5 years from the recognition of cirrhosis[4] and is accompanied by a significant decrease in survival to less than 35% at 5 years.[5,6] For further details on the natural history of chronic HBV infection, see the article by McMahon elsewhere in this issue.

ANTIVIRAL THERAPY IN ADVANCED CHRONIC HEPATITIS B

Therapeutic goals in the patient with chronic HBV with cirrhosis include complete viral suppression, sustained HBeAg seroconversion (where applicable), the prevention or even reversal of hepatic decompensation, reduction of HCC risk, and prevention of viral recurrence after transplantation. Large-scale studies with adequate follow-up periods have confirmed a relationship between viral replication (reflected in serum HBV DNA levels) and development of cirrhosis[7] and HCC.[8] Further results and implications of the Taiwanese REVEAL study are described in the article by McMahon elsewhere in this issue. Detectable viremia before liver transplantation (OLT) is associated with reduced patient and graft survival because of HBV recurrence in the graft,[9–13] underscoring the importance of achieving viral suppression before OLT.

Antiviral therapy is indicated in all cirrhotic patients with evidence of active HBV viral replication (HBV DNA >2000 IU/mL), regardless of alanine aminotransferase (ALT)

[a] Department of Gastroenterology & Hepatology, Singapore General Hospital, Outram Road, S (169608), Republic of Singapore
[b] Division of Hepatology, Schiff Liver Institute, Center for Liver Diseases, University of Miami Miller School of Medicine, 1500 NW 12 Avenue, Jackson Medical Tower E-1101, Miami, FL 33136, USA
* Corresponding author.
E-mail address: mhyhui@gmail.com

Clin Liver Dis 14 (2010) 477–493
doi:10.1016/j.cld.2010.05.006
1089-3261/10/$ – see front matter © 2010 Elsevier Inc. All rights reserved.

levels or HBeAg status.[14,15] It is also indicated in all decompensated cirrhotic patients with increased ALT levels if HBV DNA is detectable (regardless of titer).[15] Viral flares are less well tolerated in the patient with end-stage liver disease and may result in clinical deterioration or death,[16,17] hence the importance of achieving viral suppression in such patients and the importance of treatment compliance. Some investigators also advocate antiviral therapy for cirrhotic patients even in the absence of viral replication.[14] Antiviral prophylaxis with nucleos(t)ide analogues is also indicated in the aviremic patient with HBV who requires immunosuppressive or cytotoxic chemotherapy. Prophylaxis should be commenced before immunosuppressive therapy and continued throughout the course of treatment.[15,18]

Once antiviral treatment with nucleos(t)ide analogues is commenced, treatment is usually life-long in cirrhotic patients, as interruption of therapy is associated with a risk of viral reactivation, hepatic decompensation,[19,20] and histologic regression despite benefit while on therapy.[21,22]

Monotherapy and Choice of Agent

Interferon alpha-2a

Interferon alpha-2a, standard and pegylated formulations, has been approved by the US Food and Drug Administration for the treatment of chronic HBV infection. Interferon enhances host response to HBV infection, resulting indirectly in HBV clearance. Interferon directly inhibits hepatic stellate cell activation.[23] In animal models, it has been shown to reduce collagen gene transcription[24] and reverse cirrhosis.[25] Long-term studies confirm that interferon promotes viral clearance and prevents the development of cirrhosis, clinical decompensation,[26-28] and development of HCC.[29] However, its use in advanced liver disease is potentially hazardous as it may precipitate clinical decompensation, increasing the risk of bacterial infection by inducing an imminent viral flare,[30-32] even with low doses. For these reasons, interferon therapy in decompensated HBV cirrhosis is contraindicated.[14,15] In the well-compensated HBV cirrhotic patient, however, there was no difference in the need for dose reduction or discontinuation of interferon therapy compared with noncirrhotic patients.[33] Also, registration trials for pegylated interferon alpha-2a did not result in hepatic decompensation despite advanced fibrosis in some subjects,[34-36] although viral flares with ALT levels increased more than 5 times the upper limit of normal were reported, suggesting that there may be a role for pegylated interferon in well-compensated cirrhosis.[14]

Nucleos(t)ide analogues

Nucleoside (lamivudine, entecavir, telbivudine) and nucleotide (adefovir dipivoxil, tenofovir disoproxil fumarate) analogues of the HBV DNA polymerase are approved for chronic HBV therapy in the United States and elsewhere. Nucleos(t)ide analogues have shown benefits in delaying disease progression, stabilizing or even reversing hepatic decompensation, promoting histologic improvement,[37-39] and salvaging patients with decompensated HBV disease.[40-42] Nucleos(t)ide analogues have the advantage of profound viral suppression and safety, even in decompensated cirrhosis. Since their introduction, the number of candidates listed for OLT for decompensated cirrhosis caused by HBV in the United States has fallen significantly.[11]

Lamivudine was the first licensed oral agent studied in advanced liver disease. Studies have demonstrated effective viral suppression, prevention of disease progression in advanced fibrosis,[43] survival benefit,[41] and improved clinical outcomes reducing the need for OLT.[44-47] However, in view of its resistance profile (70% drug resistance at 5 years),[48] lamivudine monotherapy is no longer the treatment of choice for patients with chronic HBV.[14,15]

Entecavir is the current nucleoside analogue of choice for chronic HBV treatment. Studies have demonstrated high potency and good safety.[49,50] It has a high genetic barrier to resistance in treatment-naive patients[51] (1.2% viral resistance cumulative for up to 6 years of treatment). However, this advantage is lost in the presence of lamivudine resistance, as 7% of patients treated with entecavir monotherapy develop cross-resistance to entecavir within 1 year of initiation of treatment and up to 51% after 5 years.[51] Studies of its safety and efficacy in advanced cirrhosis are ongoing. In a recent study of 16 consecutive patients, lactic acidosis (lactate 40–200 mg/dL; pH 7.02–7.35) developed in 5 patients between day 4 and 240 of entecavir therapy (3 patients with severe acidosis pH <7.3; 2 patients with compensated acidosis), all of whom had highly impaired baseline liver functions (Mayo End-stage Liver Disease [MELD] score ≥20). Lactic acidosis did not occur in patients with a MELD score of 18 or less.[52] This apparent toxicity had not been recognized previously as entecavir had shown little evidence of mitochondrial toxicity even at concentrations exceeding 100 times the maximum concentration seen in humans.[53] In contrast, other investigators who randomized 112 patients with decompensated liver disease (Child-Pugh-Turcotte score ≥7) to receive tenofovir/emtricitabine plus tenofovir/entecavir (45:45:22) found no difference in tolerability between the 3 treatment groups to week 48 and there were no unexpected safety signals during the study.[54] Similarly, a study of entecavir 1 mg versus adefovir 10 mg daily in 190 decompensated HBV patients (Child-Pugh-Turcotte score ≥7) found treatment to be well tolerated and safety results were comparable in both groups. However, entecavir had superior antiviral activity to adefovir by week 24 of treatment.[55]

Although telbivudine shares cross-resistance with lamivudine,[56] it is more potent than lamivudine in the treatment of HBeAg-positive and HBeAg-negative chronic HBV infection.[57] Its high rate of resistance (5% after 1 year of treatment; 25% after 2 years of treatment)[56] has limited its role in the treatment of chronic HBV. There are limited data on telbivudine in decompensated cirrhosis, although intuitively, its resistance profile makes it a less-than-ideal drug in this patient population.

Adefovir was the first nucleotide analogue to be approved. In studies of cirrhotic patients with lamivudine resistance, it demonstrated viral suppression, improved clinical parameters, with diminished MELD scores, and successful removal from OLT waiting lists in some cases.[58] Improved patient survival even in Child B or C cirrhotic patients was observed.[59] Although less potent, it has a better resistance profile than lamivudine (30% drug resistance at 5 years), with resistance emerging mainly in patients who do not achieve viral suppression within 48 weeks of starting therapy.[22] Adefovir has no cross-resistance with lamivudine or other nucleoside analogues, hence, its efficacy in the treatment of lamivudine-resistant chronic HBV,[60,61] before and after OLT.[58]

Tenofovir, the second nucleotide to be approved for HBV therapy, is more potent and has a better safety profile than adefovir.[62] It is effective as monotherapy or in combination (eg, with emtricitabine) in the treatment of HBV monoinfection, HBV/human immunodeficiency virus (HIV) coinfection, or lamivudine-resistant HBV.[62–64] Although less nephrotoxic than adefovir, instances of nephropathy have been reported in patients with HIV who were treated with tenofovir for extended periods.[65–69] There are only limited data on its use in decompensated cirrhosis with case reports describing patients with lamivudine resistance or adefovir resistance deriving clinical benefit when salvaged with tenofovir.[70,71] As mentioned earlier, a recent study that randomized 112 patients with decompensated liver disease (Child-Pugh-Turcotte score ≥7) to receive tenofovir, emtricitabine plus tenofovir, or entecavir found no difference in tolerability with the 3 regimens to week 48 and no unexpected toxicity.[54] A multicenter European study enrolled 39 patients with chronic HBV with advanced liver disease and hepatic fibrosis with combination entecavir-tenofovir rescue treatment (median treatment duration 10.5 months) for multidrug-resistant HBV. Cirrhotic patients in this study did not develop clinical decompensation and rescue therapy was found to be safe, efficient, and well tolerated.[72] A sub-analysis of the tenofovir registration trials GS-174-0102 (HBeAg-negative patients) and GS-174-0103 (HBeAg-positive patients) compared treatment outcomes among enrolled patients with cirrhosis versus noncirrhotic patients for 96 weeks of therapy. Tenofovir efficacy and safety were comparable in cirrhotic and noncirrhotic patients with good tolerability.[73] Data on tenofovir resistance are limited.[74,75] Of the 426 patients who received tenofovir in the registration trials, only 2 patients developed mutations of the reverse transcriptase domain of HBV polymerase.[62] Neither patient had virologic breakthrough; phenotypic studies showed full susceptibility to tenofovir or a nonviable, nonreplicative virus in cell culture.

The topic of drug resistance in antiviral HBV therapy is covered in greater detail in the article by Locarnini and Bowden elsewhere in this issue. Agents with high barriers to resistance (eg, entecavir, tenofovir) should be considered as first-line therapy,[76] especially in the HBV patient with end-stage liver disease.

Patients with cirrhosis are also at risk of acute kidney injury for various reasons, including hepatorenal syndrome,[77] and doses of all nucleos(t)ide analogues must be adjusted according to creatinine clearance as appropriate.

Combination Therapy Versus Sequential Monotherapy

There are no formal guidelines to guide combination nucleoside-nucleotide therapy in the treatment-naive cirrhotic patient with chronic HBV. There is also no evidence to date that combination regimens produce higher rates of HBeAg seroconversion, more rapid declines in serum HBV DNA levels, or more rapid clinical improvements than monotherapy in the decompensated HBV cirrhotic patient.[76,78] Some investigators advise this combination as first-line therapy in decompensated patients to obviate the development of drug resistance.[14] However, definitive studies of combination therapy are required in this patient population. Patients receiving combination therapy for established drug resistance should be maintained on both drugs indefinitely as the withdrawal of one or both drugs may precipitate a viral flare.

The combination of dual nucleoside-nucleoside analogue therapy has not demonstrated added benefit in chronic HBV therapy perhaps because both agents compete for phosphorylation by cellular kinases and nucleosides of the same structural group share the same profiles of resistant mutations.[79–81]

In the past, sequential monotherapy was used in patients who developed resistance to lamivudine by switching them to adefovir therapy with a short overlap period of 2 to 3 months.[82] However, studies have suggested that switching from lamivudine to adefovir is associated with accelerated adefovir resistance.[83–85] This strategy has been replaced with add-on combination therapy instead,[14,15] which has confirmed viral suppression without long-term resistance to adefovir when the latter is added to lamivudine in the presence of lamivudine resistance.[86] The European Association for the Study of the Liver (EASL) guidelines recommend the addition of a second drug without cross-resistance if HBV DNA is still detectable by week 48 of initial therapy.[87]

MONITORING THE HBV PATIENT WITH CIRRHOSIS

The emergence of drug resistance is poorly tolerated in patients with end-stage liver disease. Cirrhotic patients on antiviral treatment should be monitored regularly for this event, as discussed in the articles by Lok and Locarnini elsewhere in this issue. Antiviral failure (caused by resistance) in HBV patients awaiting transplant was not found to impair clinical outcomes if recognized early and when salvage therapy was initiated promptly.[88]

Patients with cirrhosis are at high risk for developing HCC and other complications. Timely surveillance for HCC, varices,[89] prophylaxis against spontaneous bacterial peritonitis,[90–92] and early diagnosis of hepatic encephalopathy can delay life-threatening complications, reduce the need for hospitalization, and potentially improve survival pending liver transplantation.[93]

The American Association for the Study of Liver Diseases recommends HCC surveillance for the HBV cirrhotic patient with 6 to 12 monthly ultrasound examinations alone or in combination with measurement of α-fetoprotein levels, or with α-fetoprotein levels alone where ultrasound facilities are not available.[15] This approach has been endorsed by other authorities.[14] Studies of HCC diagnosis generally indicate 60% sensitivity and 90% specificity for liver ultrasound[94] and a much lower sensitivity (25%–65%) for α-fetoprotein levels alone. In patients undergoing HCC surveillance while awaiting liver transplantation, multiphasic computed tomography or magnetic resonance imaging is associated with the greatest gain in life expectancy and is possibly cost-effective as well. Caution should be exercised on contrast-induced nephrotoxicity in these patients with end-stage liver disease.[95,96]

HBV patients with overtly decompensated cirrhosis should be referred to a transplant center, although, as discussed earlier, antiviral therapy may abort or even reverse progression of hepatic decompensation.

HBV PROPHYLAXIS AFTER OLT

By the early 1990s, HBV infection was considered a relative contraindication to OLT in view of near universal recurrence of HBV infection and more rapid disease progression after OLT in the graft,[97,98] including the development of fibrosing cholestatic hepatitis, a form of hepatitis that is usually fatal. With the availability of HBV immunoprophylaxis and antiviral therapy, the outcomes of OLT for end-stage HBV disease are now similar to or better than that for other indications.[9,99,100] The aim of HBV treatment in the pre-OLT candidate is to suppress HBV DNA to the lowest possible level before transplantation.[59,101,102] High HBV DNA levels pre-OLT (regardless of wild-type or drug-resistance mutation) increase the risk of post-OLT prophylaxis failure.[12,13]

Hepatitis B Immunoglobulin

The introduction of passive immune prophylaxis with hepatitis B Immunoglobulin (HBIG) was the key initial step in reducing the rate of HBV reinfection after OLT. Protective mechanisms of HBIG include binding to circulating virions, binding to hepatocyte HBV receptor and promoting antibody-dependent cell-mediated cytotoxicity with cell lysis.[103] HBIG protects against HBV reinfection irrespective of the viral subtype.[104] In 1991, a study of 334 patients by Samuel and colleagues[105] reported the prevention of HBV recurrence in two-thirds of patients who had received at least 6 months of HBIG after OLT. Multiple other studies later confirmed the efficacy of HBIG therapy.[106–108] However, there are considerable limitations to its use, including cost, the inconvenience of regular infusions, and a lack of data to guide optimal dosing and treatment duration. Currently, most prophylactic regimens involve administration of high-dose (10,000 IU) intravenous HBIG in the anhepatic phase, followed by daily intravenous HBIG for a week. The subsequent dosing regimen varies by center. Fixed and variable dosing schedules as well as intravenous or intramuscular routes have been used. To date, there are no prospective controlled trials to guide the optimal dose of HBIG or the minimum level of anti-HBs required to prevent graft reinfection. Some centers have also successfully used fixed-dose monthly regimens to prevent HBV recurrence, rather than titrating the dose to achieve specific anti-HBs titers.[98]

To circumvent the inconvenience of regular HBIG infusions, centers have explored the efficacy of alternative routes of administration, such as intramuscular injections. More recent data indicate that regardless of the route of injection, circulating levels of anti-HBs are equivalent, especially when HBIG is used in combination with oral antiviral therapy.[109]

HBV recurrence despite HBIG prophylaxis reflects inadequate protective levels of anti-HBs or a pre-S/S mutation with a conformational change in the "a" moiety of the S antigen, impairing HBV binding to the HBIG site.[110] The development of such an escape mutation has been associated with poor clinical outcomes and progression to graft failure.[111]

Combination HBIG-Antiviral Prophylaxis

High HBV recurrence rates with HBIG or lamivudine monotherapy[46] led to combination therapy with lamivudine and HBIG to prevent graft reinfection. Meta-analyses have confirmed the benefit of combination HBIG-lamivudine prophylaxis for the prevention of HBV recurrence, HBV-related death, and all-cause mortality.[112] This combination has had the greatest effect on reducing HBV recurrence after OLT, which has now become an uncommon event.[99,112–116] The use of HBIG after OLT in combination with life-long nucleoside analogues (started before or at the time of OLT) is presently the standard of care in preventing graft reinfection.[9]

Any nucleos(t)ide analogues commenced before transplant should be continued in combination with HBIG after OLT, and this has enabled the use of even lower doses of HBIG than used in previous studies.[117] In the study by Gane and colleagues,[117] intramuscular HBIG 400 or 800 IU was administered daily for the first postoperative week, then weekly in the first month and monthly thereafter. Lamivudine started before OLT was continued into the postoperative period. Lamivudine resistance had developed in all 5 patients with HBV recurrence, with a HBV recurrence rate of 1% at 1 year and 4% at 5 years. Baseline high HBV DNA titer greater than 10^7 copies/mL was the key predictor of viral recurrence. More effective antiviral therapy initiated before OLT may therefore reduce the risk of HBV recurrence if the viral load is adequately suppressed; suggesting that the most potent regimen should be used before OLT to render the patient aviremic. Unlike earlier studies, the study by Gane and colleague[117] implied that HBIG prophylaxis need not necessarily be intravenous, even in the initial postoperative period. Other studies have demonstrated pre-OLT HBV DNA levels to be inversely related to anti-HBs titers achieved after OLT; and lower anti-HBs titers associated with HBV recurrence.[118–120] These results have led to recommendations that patients at low risk for HBV recurrence (ie, HBV DNA <10,000 IU/mL) and who have wild-type HBV may be candidates for lower-dose HBIG regimens and monotherapy with nucleoside analogues. Conversely, those with high levels of HBV DNA ($\geq$20,000 IU/mL) and/or with drug-resistant HBV mutations should receive long-term HBIG and potent antivirals targeted at the resistant strain.[121]

Adefovir therapy is effective in suppressing wild-type HBV and lamivudine-resistant HBV mutants in the post-OLT patient.[58] There is little controlled data about the use of newer nucleoside analogues (eg, entecavir, emtricitabine, tenofovir, telbivudine) in the post-OLT setting, although they are effective against wild-type and lamivudine-resistant mutants in the nontransplant setting.

With the current potency of oral antiviral agents and the use of appropriate HBIG dosing, fibrosing cholestatic hepatitis is now an extremely rare form of recurrence of HBV after OLT and should not be seen unless there is patient noncompliance.

The favorable results of combination immunoprophylactic therapy challenges indefinite HBIG prophylaxis, suggesting HBIG may be withdrawn after a period of induction. Some studies have shown that in patients with low viral replication before transplant, HBIG can be discontinued after a period of combination therapy.[122,123] Yoshida and colleagues[124] reported that patients with nonreplicative HBV who received lamivudine at the time of OLT could achieve adequate immunoprophylaxis with lamivudine mono-therapy, obviating the need for HBIG. However, most of these studies were small with short follow-up periods, although HBIG is increasingly being used for a finite duration after OLT with long-term prophylaxis provided by an oral agent.

THERAPEUTIC VACCINATION IN HBV OLT RECIPIENTS

Active immunoprophylaxis is a potential strategy for the HBV transplant recipient and the HBV-naive recipient of an anti-HBc positive liver graft. If effective, it offers the possibility of protection without the use of long-term HBIG or antivirals. Unfortunately, decompensated cirrhotic patients are known to have a poorer antibody response to HBV vaccination, regardless of the underlying cause of their cirrhosis.[125]

In the post-OLT setting, vaccination attempts have produced variable results. Use of standard vaccination regimens as an adjunct to immunoprophylaxis in HBV recipients has not resulted in substantial or sustained antibody production, nor has it replaced the use of HBIG.[126] In 17 responders with anti-HBs levels ranging from 10 to 100 IU/L, HBIG was withdrawn after vaccination and 82% of patients remained free of infection (defined as negative serum HBsAg and HBV DNA) after a median follow-up of 14 months.[127] All patients were aviremic before liver transplantation and none were concurrently treated with oral antiviral therapy. However, in a report of 52 Chinese patients, 2 courses of double-dose recombinant HBV vaccine with unlimited lamivudine provided only 8% efficacy, as anti-HBs (range 12–103 IU/L) decreased rapidly even among responders.[128] Recombinant HBV vaccine has also been used in combination with new adjuvants (eg, monophosphoryl lipid A and *Quillaja saponaria*) to enhance the immunogenicity of HBV vaccines. An early report on 10 patients produced encouraging results, with anti-HBs titers achieved greater than 500 IU/L enabling HBIG to be withdrawn a year after vaccination among 5 responders.[129] Common features of OLT recipients included in vaccination studies were undetectable serum HBV DNA before OLT, prolonged period of time from OLT to vaccination, low doses of maintenance immunosuppression, and serum HBV DNA negative by polymerase chain reaction (PCR) at the start of vaccination.[9] These results provide proof-of-principle that HBV vaccination can generate anti-HBs despite immunosuppressants in OLT recipients.

Active immunoprophylaxis remains a promising strategy for post-OLT patients, although further studies are needed before its use can be advocated outside clinical trials.

MANAGEMENT OF OCCULT HBV INFECTION

Occult HBV infection is defined as the presence of hepatic HBV DNA in HBsAg-negative individuals.[130] Such individuals may be seropositive or seronegative for anti-HBc and serum HBV DNA may (titers <200 IU/mL) or may not be detectable.

Persistent occult HBV infection is caused by the persistence of HBV covalently closed circular DNA within hepatocytes.[131–137] Expert opinion has defined the gold standard for occult HBV testing to be the analysis of DNA extracts from liver and blood samples by PCR, and the use of oligonucleotide primers specific for different HBV genomic regions and complementary to highly conserved nucleotide sequences.[130–132,138,139]

In occult HBV, the virus maintains the capacity to integrate into the host's genome, retaining its oncogenic potential. Several studies suggested that occult HBV may be a risk factor for cirrhosis and HCC development.[131,139–143] However, more data are required before recommendations can be made with regard to HCC surveillance or antiviral treatment in this population. Several mutations in the viral genome of patients with occult HBV infection have also been reported,[144–147] although definitive evidence of a pathogenic role for these is lacking.[148]

Patients with occult HBV receiving systemic chemo-, radio- or immunotherapy are potentially at risk of HBV reactivation,[132,149–154] although the actual risk is not yet quantified. Antiviral prophylaxis may be reasonable to prevent HBV reactivation in individuals with occult HBV who require repeated or protracted cytotoxic or immunosuppressive therapy.

Grafts from donors with occult HBV can efficiently transmit HBV infection in OLT, especially if the recipient lacks HBV antibodies, with reported frequencies of transmission ranging from 33% to 100%, especially with serum anti-HBc positive donor grafts.[98,155–160] Studies have shown that recipients positive for anti-HBc and/or anti-HBs antibodies have a lower risk of HBV acquisition, supporting vaccination of HBV-naive candidates before OLT.[156,157,159] The use of prophylactic nucleos(t)ide analogues can prevent viral transmission to the HBV-naive recipient.[161,162] Currently, some advocate the HBV-naive recipient should receive life-long nucleos(t)ide therapy[163] to prevent the development of severe aggressive disease. HBIG may not be of any specific benefit in this setting, as the graft is already infected. The use of such isolated anti-HBc positive grafts to expand the donor pool should ideally be reserved first for HBsAg-positive recipients, in whom long-term antiviral therapy is already indicated, and second for anti-HBs antibody-positive recipients.[9] However, their use may be sanctioned in HBV seronegative recipients who might not otherwise receive a graft before succumbing to their liver disease.

SUMMARY

HBV patients with overtly decompensated cirrhosis should be referred to a transplant center. The advent of nucleos(t)ide analogues has altered the natural history of HBV patients with advanced liver disease. Their combination with HBIG significantly increases patient and graft survival after OLT. Further research is required to define the optimal antiviral treatment agent, regime, and duration before and after OLT. Circumstantial evidence for an improved outcome with antiviral therapy on the natural history of HBV is the reduction in the number of patients listed for liver transplantation in the United States in the decade since licensing of lamivudine.[11]

REFERENCES

1. McMahon BJ. Epidemiology and natural history of hepatitis B. Semin Liver Dis 2005;25(Suppl 1):3–8.
2. Lavanchy D. Hepatitis B virus epidemiology, disease burden, treatment, and current and emerging prevention and control measures. J Viral Hepat 2004; 11:97–107.
3. Lok AS. Chronic hepatitis B. N Engl J Med 2002;346:1682–3.

4. Chu CM, Liaw YF. Hepatitis B virus-related cirrhosis: natural history and treatment. Semin Liver Dis 2006;26:142–52.
5. de Jongh FE, Janssen HL, de Man RA, et al. Survival and prognostic indicators in hepatitis B surface antigen-positive cirrhosis of the liver. Gastroenterology 1992;103:1630–5.
6. Fattovich G, Giustina G, Schalm SW, et al. Occurrence of hepatocellular carcinoma and decompensation in western European patients with cirrhosis type B. The EUROHEP Study Group on hepatitis B virus and cirrhosis. Hepatology 1995;21:77–82.
7. Iloeje UH, Yang HI, Su J, et al. Predicting cirrhosis risk based on the level of circulating hepatitis B viral load. Gastroenterology 2006;130:678–86.
8. Chen CJ, Yang HI, Su J, et al. Risk of hepatocellular carcinoma across a biological gradient of serum hepatitis B virus DNA level. JAMA 2006;295:65–73.
9. Terrault N, Roche B, Samuel D. Management of the hepatitis B virus in the liver transplantation setting: a European and an American perspective. Liver Transpl 2005;11:716–32.
10. Samuel D, Muller R, Alexander G, et al. Liver transplantation in European patients with the hepatitis B surface antigen. N Engl J Med 1993;329:1842–7.
11. Kim WR, Terrault NA, Pedersen RA, et al. Trends in waiting list registration for liver transplantation for viral hepatitis in the United States. Gastroenterology 2009;137:1680–6.
12. Rosenau J, Bahr MJ, Tillmann HL, et al. Lamivudine and low-dose hepatitis B immune globulin for prophylaxis of hepatitis B reinfection after liver transplantation possible role of mutations in the YMDD motif prior to transplantation as a risk factor for reinfection. J Hepatol 2001;34:895–902.
13. Seehofer D, Rayes N, Naumann U, et al. Preoperative antiviral treatment and postoperative prophylaxis in HBV-DNA positive patients undergoing liver transplantation. Transplantation 2001;72:1381–5.
14. Keeffe EB, Dieterich DT, Han SH, et al. A treatment algorithm for the management of chronic hepatitis B virus infection in the United States: 2008 update. Clin Gastroenterol Hepatol 2008;6:1315–41 [quiz: 1286].
15. Lok ASF, McMahon BJ. AASLD practice guidelines. Chronic hepatitis B: update 2009. Available at: www.aasld.org. Accessed June 2, 2010.
16. Chien RN, Lin CH, Liaw YF. The effect of lamivudine therapy in hepatic decompensation during acute exacerbation of chronic hepatitis B. J Hepatol 2003;38:322–7.
17. Tsubota A, Arase Y, Suzuki Y, et al. Lamivudine monotherapy for spontaneous severe acute exacerbation of chronic hepatitis B. J Gastroenterol Hepatol 2005;20:426–32.
18. Sorrell MF, Belongia EA, Costa J, et al. National Institutes of Health Consensus Development Conference Statement: management of hepatitis B. Ann Intern Med 2009;150:104–10.
19. Lim SG, Wai CT, Rajnakova A, et al. Fatal hepatitis B reactivation following discontinuation of nucleoside analogues for chronic hepatitis B. Gut 2002;51:597–9.
20. Zhang JM, Wang XY, Huang YX, et al. Fatal liver failure with the emergence of hepatitis B surface antigen variants with multiple stop mutations after discontinuation of lamivudine therapy. J Med Virol 2006;78:324–8.
21. Hadziyannis SJ, Tassopoulos NC, Heathcote EJ, et al. Adefovir dipivoxil for the treatment of hepatitis B e antigen-negative chronic hepatitis B. N Engl J Med 2003;348:800–7.

22. Hadziyannis SJ, Tassopoulos NC, Heathcote EJ, et al. Long-term therapy with adefovir dipivoxil for HBeAg-negative chronic hepatitis B for up to 5 years. Gastroenterology 2006;131:1743–51.

23. Bataller R, Brenner DA. Liver fibrosis. J Clin Invest 2005;115:209–18.

24. Inagaki Y, Nemoto T, Kushida M, et al. Interferon alfa down-regulates collagen gene transcription and suppresses experimental hepatic fibrosis in mice. Hepatology 2003;38:890–9.

25. Matthew TC, Abdeen S, Dashti H, et al. Effect of alpha-interferon and alpha-tocopherol in reversing hepatic cirrhosis in rats. Anat Histol Embryol 2007;36:88–93.

26. Niederau C, Heintges T, Lange S, et al. Long-term follow-up of HBeAg-positive patients treated with interferon alfa for chronic hepatitis B. N Engl J Med 1996;334:1422–7.

27. Fattovich G, Giustina G, Realdi G, et al. Long-term outcome of hepatitis B e antigen-positive patients with compensated cirrhosis treated with interferon alfa. European Concerted Action on Viral Hepatitis (EUROHEP). Hepatology 1997;26:1338–42.

28. Lau DT, Everhart J, Kleiner DE, et al. Long-term follow-up of patients with chronic hepatitis B treated with interferon alfa. Gastroenterology 1997;113:1660–7.

29. Lin SM, Yu ML, Lee CM, et al. Interferon therapy in HBeAg positive chronic hepatitis reduces progression to cirrhosis and hepatocellular carcinoma. J Hepatol 2007;46:45–52.

30. Hoofnagle JH, Di Bisceglie AM, Waggoner JG, et al. Interferon alfa for patients with clinically apparent cirrhosis due to chronic hepatitis B. Gastroenterology 1993;104:1116–21.

31. Marcellin P, Giuily N, Loriot MA, et al. Prolonged interferon-alpha therapy of hepatitis B virus-related decompensated cirrhosis. J Viral Hepat 1997;4(Suppl 1):21–6.

32. Perrillo R, Tamburro C, Regenstein F, et al. Low-dose, titratable interferon alfa in decompensated liver disease caused by chronic infection with hepatitis B virus. Gastroenterology 1995;109:908–16.

33. Buster EH, Hansen BE, Buti M, et al. Peginterferon alpha-2b is safe and effective in HBeAg-positive chronic hepatitis B patients with advanced fibrosis. Hepatology 2007;46:388–94.

34. Lau GK, Piratvisuth T, Luo KX, et al. Peginterferon alfa-2a, lamivudine, and the combination for HBeAg-positive chronic hepatitis B. N Engl J Med 2005;352:2682–95.

35. Marcellin P, Lau GK, Bonino F, et al. Peginterferon alfa-2a alone, lamivudine alone, and the two in combination in patients with HBeAg-negative chronic hepatitis B. N Engl J Med 2004;351:1206–17.

36. Marcellin P, Lau GK, Zeuzem S, et al. Comparing the safety, tolerability and quality of life in patients with chronic hepatitis B vs chronic hepatitis C treated with peginterferon alpha-2a. Liver Int 2008;28:477–85.

37. Lai CL, Chien RN, Leung NW, et al. A one-year trial of lamivudine for chronic hepatitis B. Asia Hepatitis Lamivudine Study Group. N Engl J Med 1998;339:61–8.

38. Suzuki Y, Kumada H, Ikeda K, et al. Histological changes in liver biopsies after one year of lamivudine treatment in patients with chronic hepatitis B infection. J Hepatol 1999;30:743–8.

39. Dienstag JL, Schiff ER, Wright TL, et al. Lamivudine as initial treatment for chronic hepatitis B in the United States. N Engl J Med 1999;341:1256–63.

40. Yao FY, Bass NM. Lamivudine treatment in patients with severely decompensated cirrhosis due to replicating hepatitis B infection. J Hepatol 2000;33:301–7.

41. Yao FY, Terrault NA, Freise C, et al. Lamivudine treatment is beneficial in patients with severely decompensated cirrhosis and actively replicating hepatitis B infection awaiting liver transplantation: a comparative study using a matched, untreated cohort. Hepatology 2001;34:411–6.

42. Fontana RJ, Keeffe EB, Carey W, et al. Effect of lamivudine treatment on survival of 309 North American patients awaiting liver transplantation for chronic hepatitis B. Liver Transpl 2002;8:433–9.

43. Liaw YF, Sung JJ, Chow WC, et al. Lamivudine for patients with chronic hepatitis B and advanced liver disease. N Engl J Med 2004;351:1521–31.

44. Villeneuve JP, Condreay LD, Willems B, et al. Lamivudine treatment for decompensated cirrhosis resulting from chronic hepatitis B. Hepatology 2000;31:207–10.

45. Kapoor D, Guptan RC, Wakil SM, et al. Beneficial effects of lamivudine in hepatitis B virus-related decompensated cirrhosis. J Hepatol 2000;33:308–12.

46. Perrillo RP, Wright T, Rakela J, et al. A multicenter United States-Canadian trial to assess lamivudine monotherapy before and after liver transplantation for chronic hepatitis B. Hepatology 2001;33:424–32.

47. Hann HW, Fontana RJ, Wright T, et al. A United States compassionate use study of lamivudine treatment in nontransplantation candidates with decompensated hepatitis B virus-related cirrhosis. Liver Transpl 2003;9:49–56.

48. Chang TT, Lai CL, Chien RN, et al. Four years of lamivudine treatment in Chinese patients with chronic hepatitis B. J Gastroenterol Hepatol 2004;19:1276–82.

49. Chang TT, Gish RG, de Man R, et al. A comparison of entecavir and lamivudine for HBeAg-positive chronic hepatitis B. N Engl J Med 2006;354:1001–10.

50. Lai CL, Shouval D, Lok AS, et al. Entecavir versus lamivudine for patients with HBeAg-negative chronic hepatitis B. N Engl J Med 2006;354:1011–20.

51. Tenney DJ, Rose RE, Baldick CJ, et al. Long-term monitoring shows hepatitis B virus resistance to entecavir in nucleoside-naive patients is rare through 5 years of therapy. Hepatology 2009;49:1503–14.

52. Lange CM, Bojunga J, Hofmann WP, et al. Severe lactic acidosis during treatment of chronic hepatitis B with entecavir in patients with impaired liver function. Hepatology 2009;50:2001–6.

53. Mazzucco CE, Hamatake RK, Colonno RJ, et al. Entecavir for treatment of hepatitis B virus displays no in vitro mitochondrial toxicity or DNA polymerase gamma inhibition. Antimicrob Agents Chemother 2008;52:598–605.

54. Liaw YF, Lee CM, Akarca US, et al. Interim results of a double-blind, randomized phase 2 study of the safety of tenofovir disoproxil fumarate, emtricitabine plus tenofovir disoproxil fumarate, and entecavir in the treatment of chronic hepatitis B subjects with decompensated liver disease. Hepatology 2009;50:409A.

55. Liaw YF, Raptopoulou-Gigi M, Cheinquer H, et al. Efficacy and safety of entecavir versus adefovir in chronic hepatitis B patients with evidence of hepatic decompensation. Hepatology 2009;50:505A.

56. Liaw YF, Gane E, Leung N, et al. 2-Year GLOBE trial results: telbivudine is superior to lamivudine in patients with chronic hepatitis B. Gastroenterology 2009;136:486–95.

57. Lai CL, Gane E, Liaw YF, et al. Telbivudine versus lamivudine in patients with chronic hepatitis B. N Engl J Med 2007;357:2576–88.

58. Schiff ER, Lai CL, Hadziyannis S, et al. Adefovir dipivoxil therapy for lamivudine-resistant hepatitis B in pre- and post-liver transplantation patients. Hepatology 2003;38:1419–27.

59. Schiff E, Lai CL, Hadziyannis S, et al. Adefovir dipivoxil for wait-listed and post-liver transplantation patients with lamivudine-resistant hepatitis B: final long-term results. Liver Transpl 2007;13:349–60.

60. Perrillo R, Hann HW, Mutimer D, et al. Adefovir dipivoxil added to ongoing lamivudine in chronic hepatitis B with YMDD mutant hepatitis B virus. Gastroenterology 2004;126:81–90.

61. Peters MG, Hann Hw H, Martin P, et al. Adefovir dipivoxil alone or in combination with lamivudine in patients with lamivudine-resistant chronic hepatitis B. Gastroenterology 2004;126:91–101.

62. Marcellin P, Heathcote EJ, Buti M, et al. Tenofovir disoproxil fumarate versus adefovir dipivoxil for chronic hepatitis B. N Engl J Med 2008;359:2442–55.

63. Kuo A, Dienstag JL, Chung RT. Tenofovir disoproxil fumarate for the treatment of lamivudine-resistant hepatitis B. Clin Gastroenterol Hepatol 2004;2:266–72.

64. van Bommel F, Zollner B, Sarrazin C, et al. Tenofovir for patients with lamivudine-resistant hepatitis B virus (HBV) infection and high HBV DNA level during adefovir therapy. Hepatology 2006;44:318–25.

65. Verhelst D, Monge M, Meynard JL, et al. Fanconi syndrome and renal failure induced by tenofovir: a first case report. Am J Kidney Dis 2002;40:1331–3.

66. Izzedine H, Isnard-Bagnis C, Hulot JS, et al. Renal safety of tenofovir in HIV treatment-experienced patients. AIDS 2004;18:1074–6.

67. Karras A, Lafaurie M, Furco A, et al. Tenofovir-related nephrotoxicity in human immunodeficiency virus-infected patients: three cases of renal failure, Fanconi syndrome, and nephrogenic diabetes insipidus. Clin Infect Dis 2003;36:1070–3.

68. Lee JC, Marosok RD. Acute tubular necrosis in a patient receiving tenofovir. AIDS 2003;17:2543–4.

69. Coca S, Perazella MA. Rapid communication: acute renal failure associated with tenofovir: evidence of drug-induced nephrotoxicity. Am J Med Sci 2002;324:342–4.

70. Taltavull TC, Chahri N, Verdura B, et al. Successful treatment with tenofovir in a Child C cirrhotic patient with lamivudine-resistant hepatitis B virus awaiting liver transplantation. Post-transplant results. Transpl Int 2005;18:879–83.

71. Ratziu V, Thibault V, Benhamou Y, et al. Successful rescue therapy with tenofovir in a patient with hepatic decompensation and adefovir resistant HBV mutant. Comp Hepatol 2006;5:1.

72. Petersen J, Lutgehetmann M, Zoulim F, et al. Entecavir and tenofovir combination therapy in chronic hepatitis B: rescue therapy in patients with advanced fibrosis and multiple previous treatment failures. Results from an international multicenter cohort study. Hepatology 2009;50:496A.

73. Buti M, Hadziyannis SJ, Mathurin P, et al. Two years safety and efficacy of tenofovir disoproxil fumarate (TDF) in patients with HBV-induced cirrhosis. Gastroenterology 2009;136:865A.

74. Sheldon J, Camino N, Rodes B, et al. Selection of hepatitis B virus polymerase mutations in HIV-coinfected patients treated with tenofovir. Antivir Ther 2005;10:727–34.

75. Delaney WE, Ray AS, Yang H, et al. Intracellular metabolism and in vitro activity of tenofovir against hepatitis B virus. Antimicrob Agents Chemother 2006;50:2471–7.

76. Peters MG. Special populations with hepatitis B virus infection. Hepatology 2009;49:S146–55.

77. Garcia-Tsao G, Parikh CR, Viola A. Acute kidney injury in cirrhosis. Hepatology 2008;48:2064–77.

78. Sung JJ, Lai JY, Zeuzem S, et al. Lamivudine compared with lamivudine and adefovir dipivoxil for the treatment of HBeAg-positive chronic hepatitis B. J Hepatol 2008;48:728–35.

79. Lai CL, Leung N, Teo EK, et al. A 1-year trial of telbivudine, lamivudine, and the combination in patients with hepatitis B e antigen-positive chronic hepatitis B. Gastroenterology 2005;129:528–36.
80. Ghany M, Liang TJ. Drug targets and molecular mechanisms of drug resistance in chronic hepatitis B. Gastroenterology 2007;132:1574–85.
81. Locarnini S, Hatzakis A, Heathcote J, et al. Management of antiviral resistance in patients with chronic hepatitis B. Antivir Ther 2004;9:679–93.
82. Liaw YF. Rescue therapy for lamivudine-resistant chronic hepatitis B: when and how? Hepatology 2007;45:266–8.
83. Fung SK, Chae HB, Fontana RJ, et al. Virologic response and resistance to adefovir in patients with chronic hepatitis B. J Hepatol 2006;44:283–90.
84. Lee YS, Suh DJ, Lim YS, et al. Increased risk of adefovir resistance in patients with lamivudine-resistant chronic hepatitis B after 48 weeks of adefovir dipivoxil monotherapy. Hepatology 2006;43:1385–91.
85. Rapti I, Dimou E, Mitsoula P, et al. Adding-on versus switching-to adefovir therapy in lamivudine-resistant HBeAg-negative chronic hepatitis B. Hepatology 2007;45:307–13.
86. Lampertico P, Vigano M, Manenti E, et al. Low resistance to adefovir combined with lamivudine: a 3-year study of 145 lamivudine-resistant hepatitis B patients. Gastroenterology 2007;133:1445–51.
87. European Association for the Study of the Liver. EASL clinical practice guidelines: management of chronic hepatitis B. J Hepatol 2009;50:227.
88. Osborn MK, Han SH, Regev A, et al. Outcomes of patients with hepatitis B who developed antiviral resistance while on the liver transplant waiting list. Clin Gastroenterol Hepatol 2007;5:1454–61.
89. de Franchis R. Evolving consensus in portal hypertension. Report of the Baveno IV consensus workshop on methodology of diagnosis and therapy in portal hypertension. J Hepatol 2005;43:167–76.
90. Tito L, Rimola A, Gines P, et al. Recurrence of spontaneous bacterial peritonitis in cirrhosis: frequency and predictive factors. Hepatology 1988;8:27–31.
91. Gines P, Rimola A, Planas R, et al. Norfloxacin prevents spontaneous bacterial peritonitis recurrence in cirrhosis: results of a double-blind, placebo-controlled trial. Hepatology 1990;12:716–24.
92. Runyon BA. Management of adult patients with ascites due to cirrhosis: an update. Hepatology 2009;49:2087–107.
93. Grewal P, Martin P. Care of the cirrhotic patient. Clin Liver Dis 2009;13:331–40.
94. Bolondi L, Gaiani S, Gebel M. Portohepatic vascular pathology and liver disease: diagnosis and monitoring. Eur J Ultrasound 1998;7(Suppl 3): S41–52.
95. Saab S, Ly D, Nieto J, et al. Hepatocellular carcinoma screening in patients waiting for liver transplantation: a decision analytic model. Liver Transpl 2003;9: 672–81.
96. Choi D, Kim SH, Lim JH, et al. Detection of hepatocellular carcinoma: combined T2-weighted and dynamic gadolinium-enhanced MRI versus combined CT during arterial portography and CT hepatic arteriography. J Comput Assist Tomogr 2001;25:777–85.
97. O'Grady JG, Smith HM, Davies SE, et al. Hepatitis B virus reinfection after orthotopic liver transplantation. Serological and clinical implications. J Hepatol 1992; 14:104–11.
98. Mutimer D. Review article: hepatitis B and liver transplantation. Aliment Pharmacol Ther 2006;23:1031–41.

99. Han SH, Ofman J, Holt C, et al. An efficacy and cost-effectiveness analysis of combination hepatitis B immune globulin and lamivudine to prevent recurrent hepatitis B after orthotopic liver transplantation compared with hepatitis B immune globulin monotherapy. Liver Transpl 2000;6:741–8.

100. Kim WR, Poterucha JJ, Kremers WK, et al. Outcome of liver transplantation for hepatitis B in the United States. Liver Transpl 2004;10:968–74.

101. Grellier L, Mutimer D, Ahmed M, et al. Lamivudine prophylaxis against reinfection in liver transplantation for hepatitis B cirrhosis. Lancet 1996;348:1212–5.

102. Samuel D. Management of hepatitis B in liver transplantation patients. Semin Liver Dis 2004;24(Suppl 1):55–62.

103. Zuckerman JN. Review: hepatitis B immune globulin for prevention of hepatitis B infection. J Med Virol 2007;79:919–21.

104. Waters JA, Brown SE, Steward MW, et al. Analysis of the antigenic epitopes of hepatitis B surface antigen involved in the induction of a protective antibody response. Virus Res 1992;22:1–12.

105. Samuel D, Bismuth A, Mathieu D, et al. Passive immunoprophylaxis after liver transplantation in HBsAg-positive patients. Lancet 1991;337:813–5.

106. Terrault NA, Zhou S, Combs C, et al. Prophylaxis in liver transplant recipients using a fixed dosing schedule of hepatitis B immunoglobulin. Hepatology 1996;24:1327–33.

107. Rimoldi P, Belli LS, Rondinara GF, et al. Recurrent HBV/HDV infections under different immunoprophylaxis protocols. Transplant Proc 1993;25:2675–6.

108. Steinmuller T, Seehofer D, Rayes N, et al. Increasing applicability of liver transplantation for patients with hepatitis B-related liver disease. Hepatology 2002;35:1528–35.

109. Hooman N, Rifai K, Hadem J, et al. Antibody to hepatitis B surface antigen trough levels and half-lives do not differ after intravenous and intramuscular hepatitis B immunoglobulin administration after liver transplantation. Liver Transpl 2008;14:435–42.

110. Ghany MG, Ayola B, Villamil FG, et al. Hepatitis B virus S mutants in liver transplant recipients who were reinfected despite hepatitis B immune globulin prophylaxis. Hepatology 1998;27:213–22.

111. Protzer-Knolle U, Naumann U, Bartenschlager R, et al. Hepatitis B virus with antigenically altered hepatitis B surface antigen is selected by high-dose hepatitis B immune globulin after liver transplantation. Hepatology 1998;27:254–63.

112. Loomba R, Rowley AK, Wesley R, et al. Hepatitis B immunoglobulin and lamivudine improve hepatitis B-related outcomes after liver transplantation: meta-analysis. Clin Gastroenterol Hepatol 2008;6:696–700.

113. Dumortier J, Le Derf Y, Guillem P, et al. Favorable outcome of liver transplantation despite a high hepatitis B virus replication: beyond the limits? Transpl Infect Dis 2006;8:182–4.

114. Markowitz JS, Martin P, Conrad AJ, et al. Prophylaxis against hepatitis B recurrence following liver transplantation using combination lamivudine and hepatitis B immune globulin. Hepatology 1998;28:585–9.

115. Angus PW, McCaughan GW, Gane EJ, et al. Combination low-dose hepatitis B immune globulin and lamivudine therapy provides effective prophylaxis against posttransplantation hepatitis B. Liver Transpl 2000;6:429–33.

116. Marzano A, Salizzoni M, Debernardi-Venon W, et al. Prevention of hepatitis B virus recurrence after liver transplantation in cirrhotic patients treated with lamivudine and passive immunoprophylaxis. J Hepatol 2001;34:903–10.

117. Gane EJ, Angus PW, Strasser S, et al. Lamivudine plus low-dose hepatitis B immunoglobulin to prevent recurrent hepatitis B following liver transplantation. Gastroenterology 2007;132:931–7.
118. Neff GW, O'Brien CB, Nery J, et al. Outcomes in liver transplant recipients with hepatitis B virus: resistance and recurrence patterns from a large transplant center over the last decade. Liver Transpl 2004;10:1372–8.
119. Zheng S, Chen Y, Liang T, et al. Prevention of hepatitis B recurrence after liver transplantation using lamivudine or lamivudine combined with hepatitis B immunoglobulin prophylaxis. Liver Transpl 2006;12:253–8.
120. Marzano A, Gaia S, Ghisetti V, et al. Viral load at the time of liver transplantation and risk of hepatitis B virus recurrence. Liver Transpl 2005;11:402–9.
121. Coffin CS, Terrault NA. Management of hepatitis B in liver transplant recipients. J Viral Hepat 2007;14(Suppl 1):37–44.
122. Dodson SF, de Vera ME, Bonham CA, et al. Lamivudine after hepatitis B immune globulin is effective in preventing hepatitis B recurrence after liver transplantation. Liver Transpl 2000;6:434–9.
123. Terrault NA, Wright TL, Roberts JP, et al. Combined short-term hepatitis B immunoglobulin and long-term lamivudine versus HBIG monotherapy as HBV prophylaxis in liver transplant recipients. Hepatology 1998;28:389A.
124. Yoshida H, Kato T, Levi DM, et al. Lamivudine monoprophylaxis for liver transplant recipients with non-replicating hepatitis B virus infection. Clin Transplant 2007;21:166–71.
125. Chalasani N, Smallwood G, Halcomb J, et al. Is vaccination against hepatitis B infection indicated in patients waiting for or after orthotopic liver transplantation? Liver Transpl Surg 1998;4:128–32.
126. Angelico M, Di Paolo D, Trinito MO, et al. Failure of a reinforced triple course of hepatitis B vaccination in patients transplanted for HBV-related cirrhosis. Hepatology 2002;35:176–81.
127. Sanchez-Fueyo A, Rimola A, Grande L, et al. Hepatitis B immunoglobulin discontinuation followed by hepatitis B virus vaccination: a new strategy in the prophylaxis of hepatitis B virus recurrence after liver transplantation. Hepatology 2000;31:496–501.
128. Lo CM, Liu CL, Chan SC, et al. Failure of hepatitis B vaccination in patients receiving lamivudine prophylaxis after liver transplantation for chronic hepatitis B. J Hepatol 2005;43:283–7.
129. Bienzle U, Gunther M, Neuhaus R, et al. Successful hepatitis B vaccination in patients who underwent transplantation for hepatitis B virus-related cirrhosis: preliminary results. Liver Transpl 2002;8:562–4.
130. Raimondo G, Allain JP, Brunetto MR, et al. Statements from the Taormina expert meeting on occult hepatitis B virus infection. J Hepatol 2008;49:652–7.
131. Brechot C, Thiers V, Kremsdorf D, et al. Persistent hepatitis B virus infection in subjects without hepatitis B surface antigen: clinically significant or purely "occult". Hepatology 2001;34:194–203.
132. Raimondo G, Pollicino T, Cacciola I, et al. Occult hepatitis B virus infection. J Hepatol 2007;46:160–70.
133. Mason AL, Xu L, Guo L, et al. Molecular basis for persistent hepatitis B virus infection in the liver after clearance of serum hepatitis B surface antigen. Hepatology 1998;27:1736–42.
134. Marusawa H, Uemoto S, Hijikata M, et al. Latent hepatitis B virus infection in healthy individuals with antibodies to hepatitis B core antigen. Hepatology 2000;31:488–95.

135. Pollicino T, Squadrito G, Cerenzia G, et al. Hepatitis B virus maintains its pro-oncogenic properties in the case of occult HBV infection. Gastroenterology 2004;126:102–10.
136. Zoulim F. New insight on hepatitis B virus persistence from the study of intrahe-patic viral cccDNA. J Hepatol 2005;42:302–8.
137. Werle-Lapostolle B, Bowden S, Locarnini S, et al. Persistence of cccDNA during the natural history of chronic hepatitis B and decline during adefovir dipivoxil therapy. Gastroenterology 2004;126:1750–8.
138. Conjeevaram HS, Lok AS. Occult hepatitis B virus infection: a hidden menace? Hepatology 2001;34:204–6.
139. Torbenson M, Thomas DL. Occult hepatitis B. Lancet Infect Dis 2002;2:479–86.
140. Marrero JA, Lok AS. Occult hepatitis B virus infection in patients with hepatocel-lular carcinoma: innocent bystander, cofactor, or culprit? Gastroenterology 2004;126:347–50.
141. Brechot C. Pathogenesis of hepatitis B virus-related hepatocellular carcinoma: old and new paradigms. Gastroenterology 2004;127:S56–61.
142. Donato F, Gelatti U, Limina RM, et al. Southern Europe as an example of inter-action between various environmental factors: a systematic review of the epide-miologic evidence. Oncogene 2006;25:3756–70.
143. Cougot D, Neuveut C, Buendia MA. HBV induced carcinogenesis. J Clin Virol 2005;34(Suppl 1):S75–8.
144. Blum HE, Galun E, Liang TJ, et al. Naturally occurring missense mutation in the polymerase gene terminating hepatitis B virus replication. J Virol 1991;65: 1836–42.
145. Hou J, Karayiannis P, Waters J, et al. A unique insertion in the S gene of surface antigen–negative hepatitis B virus Chinese carriers. Hepatology 1995;21:273–8.
146. Kato J, Hasegawa K, Torii N, et al. A molecular analysis of viral persistence in surface antigen-negative chronic hepatitis B. Hepatology 1996;23:389–95.
147. Yamamoto K, Horikita M, Tsuda F, et al. Naturally occurring escape mutants of hepatitis B virus with various mutations in the S gene in carriers seropositive for antibody to hepatitis B surface antigen. J Virol 1994;68:2671–6.
148. Liang TJ. Hepatitis B: the virus and disease. Hepatology 2009;49:S13–21.
149. Blanpain C, Knoop C, Delforge ML, et al. Reactivation of hepatitis B after trans-plantation in patients with pre-existing anti-hepatitis B surface antigen anti-bodies: report on three cases and review of the literature. Transplantation 1998;66:883–6.
150. Lok AS, Liang RH, Chiu EK, et al. Reactivation of hepatitis B virus replication in patients receiving cytotoxic therapy. Report of a prospective study. Gastroenter-ology 1991;100:182–8.
151. Hui CK, Cheung WW, Zhang HY, et al. Kinetics and risk of de novo hepatitis B infection in HBsAg-negative patients undergoing cytotoxic chemotherapy. Gastroenterology 2006;131:59–68.
152. Loomba R, Rowley A, Wesley R, et al. Systematic review: the effect of preventive lamivudine on hepatitis B reactivation during chemotherapy. Ann Intern Med 2008;148:519–28.
153. Lalazar G, Rund D, Shouval D. Screening, prevention and treatment of viral hepatitis B reactivation in patients with haematological malignancies. Br J Haematol 2007;136:699–712.
154. Marzano A, Angelucci E, Andreone P, et al. Prophylaxis and treatment of hepa-titis B in immunocompromised patients. Dig Liver Dis 2007;39:397–408.

155. Dickson RC, Everhart JE, Lake JR, et al. Transmission of hepatitis B by transplantation of livers from donors positive for antibody to hepatitis B core antigen. The National Institute of Diabetes and Digestive and Kidney Diseases Liver Transplantation Database. Gastroenterology 1997;113:1668–74.

156. Manzarbeitia C, Reich DJ, Ortiz JA, et al. Safe use of livers from donors with positive hepatitis B core antibody. Liver Transpl 2002;8:556–61.

157. Prieto M, Gomez MD, Berenguer M, et al. De novo hepatitis B after liver transplantation from hepatitis B core antibody-positive donors in an area with high prevalence of anti-HBc positivity in the donor population. Liver Transpl 2001; 7:51–8.

158. Douglas DD, Rakela J, Wright TL, et al. The clinical course of transplantation-associated de novo hepatitis B infection in the liver transplant recipient. Liver Transpl Surg 1997;3:105–11.

159. Roque-Afonso AM, Feray C, Samuel D, et al. Antibodies to hepatitis B surface antigen prevent viral reactivation in recipients of liver grafts from anti-HBC positive donors. Gut 2002;50:95–9.

160. Roche B, Samuel D, Gigou M, et al. De novo and apparent de novo hepatitis B virus infection after liver transplantation. J Hepatol 1997;26:517–26.

161. Munoz SJ. Use of hepatitis B core antibody-positive donors for liver transplantation. Liver Transpl 2002;8:S82–7.

162. Samuel D, Forns X, Berenguer M, et al. Report of the monothematic EASL conference on liver transplantation for viral hepatitis (Paris, France, January 12–14, 2006). J Hepatol 2006;45:127–43.

163. Loss GE Jr, Mason AL, Nair S, et al. Does lamivudine prophylaxis eradicate persistent HBV DNA from allografts derived from anti-HBc-positive donors? Liver Transpl 2003;9:1258–64.

Management of Chronic Hepatitis B in Pregnancy

Corinne Buchanan, MSN, ACNP-BC, Tram T. Tran, MD*

KEYWORDS

- Hepatitis B virus • Pregnancy • Immunoprophylaxis • HBsAg

There are an estimated 350 million people who are chronically infected with the hepatitis B virus (HBV) worldwide.[1,2] HBV is a partially double-stranded DNA virus that is part of the Hepadnaviridae family.[3] The virus is transmitted vertically (mother-to-child transmission [MTCT]) and horizontally (sexual and blood products). In endemic areas, such as Asia, sub-Saharan Africa, the Pacific and Amazon basins, and regions of the Middle East, most infections occur during the perinatal period or in early childhood.[2] Infection of infants and children with HBV is also a problem in the United States; however, it varies by race and ethnicity, with the highest rate in Asian women (6%). The rates in African American, white, and Hispanic women are 1%, 0.6%, and 0.14%, respectively.[4]

In infants who are born to hepatitis B e antigen (HBeAg)–positive mothers, the risk of transmission can be as high as 70% to 90% at 6 months, and approximately 90% of these children who are exposed remain chronically infected.[2] In infants whose mothers are HBeAg positive, however, the administration of standard passive-active immunoprophylaxis with hepatitis B immunoglobulin (HBIg) and hepatitis B vaccination decreases the risk of transmission to 5% to 10%.[3] HBeAg-negative mothers carry a 10% to 40% transmission risk, and of those infants who are infected, 40% to 70% remain chronically infected.[2] As with HBeAg-positive mothers, there is also a significant decrease in transmission rates with passive-active immunoprophylaxis in those mothers who are HBeAg negative.

The hepatitis B vaccine is safe in all trimesters of pregnancy; therefore, any pregnant woman who is nonimmune should be administered the hepatitis B vaccination series. In addition to treating the mother, vaccination has the potential benefit of providing passive immunoprophylaxis to the fetus.[5] The standard vaccination strategy for infants born to mothers who test positive for hepatitis B surface antigen (HBsAg) includes the administration of 100 IU HBIg (human hepatitis B

Center for Liver Transplantation, Cedars-Sinai Medical Center, Geffen UCLA School of Medicine, 8635 West 3rd Street, Suite 590 West, Los Angeles, CA 90048, USA
* Corresponding author.
E-mail address: TranT@cshs.org

Clin Liver Dis 14 (2010) 495–504
doi:10.1016/j.cld.2010.05.008
1089-3261/10/$ – see front matter © 2010 Elsevier Inc. All rights reserved.

Immunoglobulin-VF, CSL Bioplasma) and hepatitis B vaccine (Recombivax HB [5 μg], Merck, or Engerix-B [10 μg], GlaxoSmithKline) within 12 hours of birth. The vaccination series is later completed with two additional doses (one at 4 weeks to 2 months of age and one at 6 months of age). In mothers with unknown HBsAg status at the time of birth, newborns should receive the hepatitis B vaccine within 12 hours of birth and, if subsequently found on admission screening to be HBsAg positive, newborns should then administered HBIg as soon as possible (within 7 days of birth).[6]

Perinatal transmission of HBV remains a significant cause of chronic HBV infection, despite the availability of immunoprophylaxis, and contributes to the estimated 50 million new cases of hepatitis B diagnosed annually.[7] In 2006, only 36% of all newborns received the HBV vaccine at birth in the 87 countries in which chronic HBV is endemic at a rate greater than or equal to 8% of the total population. Additionally, only 27% of all newborns globally received the hepatitis B vaccine at birth in 2006.[8]

In properly vaccinated infants whose mothers are HBsAg positive, 1% to 9% later become HBsAg positive.[9,10] Moreover, another 1% to 2% of properly vaccinated infants are unable to develop sufficient amounts of anti-HBs antibody to afford long-lasting immunity.[9] Infection, despite standard passive-active immunoprophylaxis, may be related to high levels of maternal viremia, intrauterine infection, or HBV mutation.[11–13]

TREATMENT OF HBV IN PREGNANT WOMEN

When a woman at high risk or with known HBV infection is planning on becoming pregnant, her hepatitis B status should be determined so that appropriate follow-up and a treatment plan can be determined. None of the 6 antivirals currently approved for hepatitis B are classified as Food and Drug Administration (FDA) pregnancy category A (adequate and well-controlled studies in pregnant women have failed to demonstrate a risk to the fetus in the first trimester of pregnancy, and there is no evidence of risk in later trimesters[14]).

Typically, indications for antiviral treatment within the general population are based on a combination of the following factors: elevated alanine aminotransferase, elevated serum HBV DNA, and histology of the liver tissue.[15,16] Interferon alfa-2b, lamivudine, adefovir, entecavir, peginterferon alfa-2a, telbivudine, and tenofovir are approved as initial therapy for chronic hepatitis B. Of these, the preferred first-line treatment choices for hepatitis B in the general population are peginterferon alfa-2a, entecavir, and tenofovir.[17] In women of reproductive age who are who are not planning on becoming pregnant, any of these treatments can be used as long as patients are counseled to practice contraception or abstinence to avoid contraception.[18]

There are 2 treatment principles in treating HBV during pregnancy: (1) treatment of the chronic hepatitis B (CHB) infection in the mother and (2) prevention of MTCT of HBV to the newborn. Screening of all pregnant women for HBV infection is an essential component of both principles. Routine screening with HBsAg testing in all pregnant women began in the United States in 1988. Followed by prompt immunization of newborns with standard passive-active immunoprophylaxis, screening has contributed to a decline in the incidence of CHB in the United States. The US Preventive Services Task Force recommended in 2004 that all pregnant women be screened with HBsAg testing at the first prenatal visit.[19] The current Centers for Disease Control and Prevention (CDC) HBV screening guidelines (2008) and the American College of Obstetrics and Gynecology recommend that all pregnant women be tested for HBsAg during each pregnancy and that women at high risk for CHB be screened on admission for delivery.[20,21]

Treatment of pregnant women with HBV infection is controversial because of a lack of strong evidence demonstrating the benefit of therapy. One of the major limitations is the availability of antiviral drug safety data in pregnancy. Several factors must be considered in evaluating patients for treatment of HBV during pregnancy, including the drawbacks of the treatment (eg, adverse effects, cost, and development of drug resistance). Although lacking in significant data, arguments that support treatment of HBV in pregnancy include lowering the possible complication rate from CHB in pregnancy (gestational diabetes, antepartum hemorrhage, and threatened preterm labor),[22] lowering the risk of progressive liver disease in the mother, and decreasing the risk of MTCT. Because of the limited availability of antiviral drug safety data in pregnancy, it is suggested that, if possible, antiviral treatment of pregnant women with CHB be postponed until after childbearing is complete.[17,23] For women who become pregnant while on CHB treatment, the continuation of antiviral therapy should be a decision made on careful examination of the severity of the mother's liver disease and the potential benefit versus risk to the fetus, particularly because hepatitis flares can occur after discontinuation of antiviral therapy.[17]

Decreasing Risk of MTCT

As previously discussed, maternal HBeAg status influences the risk for MTCT; HBeAg-positive mothers have a much greater risk of transmitting HBV compared with HBeAg-negative mothers (70%–90% vs 10%–40%, respectively).[2] History of threatened preterm labor, HBV in villous capillary endothelial cells, transplacental leakage of HBeAg-positive maternal blood, exposure to cervical secretions and maternal blood during labor and delivery, and specific allelic mutations in maternal HBV all may contribute to increased risk of MTCT.[4,24,25] High maternal viremia is another factor, and HBV viremia greater than 10^8 copies/mL has been correlated with MTCT risk.[10,26,27] Additionally, high HBV DNA levels have been associated with vaccine breakthrough, intrauterine infection, and HBV mutation.[6,28,29]

Many studies have been conducted with regards to maternal HBV DNA level. A 10-year meta-analysis from the Netherlands looked at 705 newborns whose mothers were HBsAg positive between 1982 and 1992. In this study, the only factor that significantly affected the protective efficacy rate of passive-active immunoprophylaxis was the maternal HBV DNA level. Whereas 100% protective efficacy was achieved in cases with maternal HBV DNA less than 150 pg/mL^{-1}, the protective efficacy rate was only 68% if the maternal HBV DNA was greater than 150 pg/mL^{-1}. Eight of the children from this meta-analysis were noted to become HBsAg positive within the first year of life. When compared with randomly chosen noninfected responders to standard passive-active immunoprophylaxis, 7 of the 8 children were noted to have significantly higher maternal HBV DNA levels before birth. This prompted the study to conclude that the extent of viremia was likely to have a large role in the failure of standard immunoprophylaxis.[30] In 1989, Ip and colleagues found similar results in which infants born to mothers with HBV DNA levels less than 150 pg/mL^{-1} were all HBsAg negative at 12 months, whereas those born to mothers with levels greater than 150 pg/mL^{-1} had a 25% to 50% chance of developing CHB regardless of immunization.[31]

A recent study in Australia examined 313 HBsAg-positive pregnant women from 2002 to 2008. Within this cohort of women, 47 were HBeAg positive and had HBV DNA viral loads greater than 10^8 copies/mL. Subsequent testing revealed that 4 of the 47 (9%) infants born to these women were HBsAg positive and HBsAb negative. All of the perinatally infected infants received the hepatitis B vaccination series, and

3 of the 4 infants received HBIg at birth. There was no perinatal transmission of HBV in any newborns (n = 91) of mothers with viral loads less than 10^8 copies/mL. This suggested that HBeAg positivity as well as maternal viral load (>10^8 copies/mL) corresponded with perinatal transmission.[10]

In HIV-infected mothers, it has been shown that administration of nucleoside analog therapy helped reduce the perinatal HIV rate from 25% to 30% to less than 2%.[32] This observation further supports the principle that higher maternal viral load contributes to higher transmission rates. It is, therefore, postulated that reduction of maternal viral load by antiviral treatment may decrease MTCT.

Antiviral Treatment in Pregnancy

The FDA has divided medications into 5 categories (A, B, C, D, and X) for use in pregnancy. Currently there are no FDA category A anti-HBV medications. There are, however, category B (animal reproduction studies have failed to demonstrate a risk to the fetus and there are no adequate and well-controlled studies in pregnant women) and category C (animal reproduction studies have shown an adverse effect on the fetus, there are no adequate and well-controlled studies in humans, and the benefits from the use of the drug in pregnant women may be acceptable despite its potential risks) options available.[14] The 6 antivirals approved for hepatitis B include adefovir dipivoxil (pregnancy category C), interferon alfa-2b (pregnancy category C), peginterferon alfa-2a (pregnancy category C), entecavir (pregnancy category C), lamivudine (pregnancy category C), tenofovir (pregnancy class B), and telbivudine (pregnancy category B).

Currently, some data are available regarding treatment during pregnancy with lamivudine and tenofovir. According to the Antiretroviral Pregnancy Registry (http://www.apregistry.com) 2009 interim report regarding antiretroviral use in pregnant women from January 1, 1989, through January 31, 2009, when a fetus is exposed to lamivudine during the first trimester of pregnancy, there is a 2.9% prevalence of birth defects (93/3226). Tenofovir demonstrated similar results with a 2.4% prevalence of birth defects (16/678).[33] These data are similar to the overall risk of birth defects in the general population.[34] Telbivudine has been shown to be safe during pregnancy with no effects on male or female fertility in animal studies; however, there are no human studies and few cases reported.[35] Interferon and peginterferon are not considered safe during pregnancy due to their antiproliferative effects.[36,37]

Most data that are available regarding lamivudine use in pregnancy are derived from the treatment of HIV-infected pregnant women throughout the course of pregnancy. Lamivudine is the second most common nucleoside used in pregnant women with HIV.[17] Studies have determined that pregnant women can safely tolerate 150-mg dosing twice a day or 300 mg dosed daily. In 1993, however, a placebo-controlled clinical trial with patients infected with CHB (median pretreatment HBV DNA level of 112 ng/L), a direct correlation was recognized between the amount of HBV DNA suppression and the dosing regimen (5, 20, 100, 300, or 600 mg daily) of lamivudine. The dosing regimen of 100 mg daily achieved 98% viral suppression, with the 2 higher daily dosages not producing any additional viral suppression.[38] Lamivudine diffuses across the placenta to fetal circulation and amniotic fluid.[39,40] There are no changes in drug pharmacokinetics secondary to pregnancy, and, therefore, it seems that lamivudine can be used in pregnancy without dosing adjustments.[39]

van Zonneveld and colleagues[41] examined 8 pregnant women with HBV DNA levels greater than 1.2×10^9 copies/mL who were treated with lamivudine (150 mg daily) starting at week 34 of pregnancy through delivery. The infants received HBIg at birth and

HBV vaccine starting at birth through 11 months. The median drop in HBV DNA levels was 98.9%. Of the 8 infants born to treated mothers, 4 were HBsAg positive at birth, but only 1 remained positive at 1 year of life. This study found that by using lamivudine the risk of perinatal transmission decreased by a factor of 2.9. No adverse effects were observed in mother or child.[41]

In a randomized, double-blind study by Xu and colleagues,[42] 150 mothers with HBV DNA greater than 1000 mEq/mL were randomized to lamivudine (100 mg daily or placebo) from week 32 of their pregnancy until 4 weeks postpartum. The newborns (n = 141) received recombinant HBV vaccine with or without HBIg. Within the group of infants who received in utero lamivudine plus passive-active immunoprophylaxis (n = 56), the frequency of HBsAg-positive infants was 10 of 56 (18%), whereas in the placebo group, in which the infants received passive-active immunization beginning at birth (n = 59), the incidence of HBsAg-positive infants was 23 of 59 (39%) (P = .014). The number of infants with detectable HBV DNA was 11 of 56 (20%) if the mothers received lamivudine compared with 27 of 59 (46%) (P = .003) in those who did not receive antiviral therapy. These data demonstrated a significant decrease in the risk of transmission when lamivudine was started in the third trimester of pregnancy.[42]

It is prudent to observe in the aforementioned study that if newborns were lost to follow-up they were considered a failure. There were more newborns in the placebo group (18/59) compared with the lamivudine group (7/56), who had missing follow-up data. Taking into account this information, without adjusting for missing data, reveals that there was not a statistically significant difference in HBsAg positivity between the 2 groups of infants (P = .368).[43]

The safety concern of the effects of antiviral therapy on the developing fetus may be partly mitigated by restricting antiviral therapy to use in the third trimester as opposed to throughout the duration of pregnancy. Other drawbacks remain, however, regarding antiviral use in pregnant patients. There are reports of lactic acidosis and hepatic steatosis in pregnant patients receiving nucleos(t)ide analogs.[1] For this reason, it is important to monitor liver enzymes and serum electrolytes if patients are to receive such treatment during pregnancy. Development of rapid and frequent drug-resistant HBV is well documented with lamivudine, and this is a particularly relevant issue in patients with high levels of HBV DNA.[36] For this reason, lamivudine is not the optimal drug of choice if a mother has an indication for a long-term CHB treatment beyond pregnancy. Acute exacerbations have also been reported after discontinuation of antiviral therapy after delivery. Withdrawal flares in the general population have been associated with discontinuation of lamivudine and occur in up to 25% of patients.[44] This is compared with 62% of patients who developed postpartum flares after receiving lamivudine during the last 4 weeks of pregnancy.[45] For this reason, women should be monitored closely after delivery for a significant increase in liver enzymes.

GENERAL RECOMMENDATIONS

Several critical issues must be addressed before recommending universal use of antiviral therapy to further reduce HBV MTCT. These include the threshold maternal HBV DNA level above which antiviral therapy would have a clear benefit, optimal timing of antiviral therapy initiation during pregnancy, choice of antiviral therapy, and duration of treatment.[43] The current strategy at this time if treatment is deemed warranted is to use lamivudine, tenofovir, or telbivudine starting at 32 weeks of pregnancy. HBV DNA level should be used in conjunction with the presence or absence of a history of perinatal transmission to determine whether or not to initiate antiviral therapy. Thus, if a previous child were HBV positive, the likelihood of perinatal transmission may be higher and subsequently the threshold serum HBV DNA level for treatment may be lower for the clinician and the mother. If the previous child were not HBV positive, however, treatment might be considered only with HBV DNA levels greater than 10^8 copies/mL (**Fig. 1**).[46]

TREATMENT OF HBV IN POSTPARTUM MOTHER AND CHILD

As discussed previously, close monitoring is necessary in the postpartum period given the higher incidence of hepatic flares. Unfortunately, many chronically infected women do not receive adequate care for their disease, particularly beyond the period of

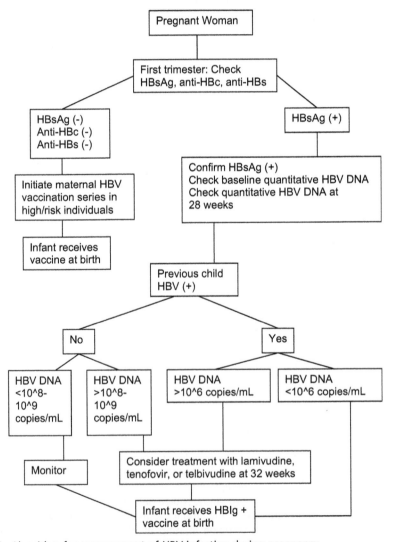

Fig. 1. Algorithm for management of HBV infection during pregnancy.

postpartum monitoring. This is especially concerning given the higher hepatocellular carcinoma rates in parous women with CHB compared with noncarriers.[47] The 6-week postpartum visit should serve as an opportunity to establish referrals for long-term medical care for CHB.

Newborns of HBsAg-positive mothers should receive HBIg and single-antigen hepatitis B vaccine within 12 hours of birth. The vaccine series should then be completed according to the recommended Advisory Committee on Immunization Practices schedule.[48] After completion of the vaccine series, testing for anti-HBs and HBsAg should be performed (typically at 9 to 18 months of age). HBsAg-negative infants with anti-HBs levels greater than 10 mIU/mL are considered protected and no further medical management is required. Conversely, those with anti-HBs levels of less than 10 mIU/mL are not adequately protected and should be revaccinated with a second 3-dose series followed by retesting 1 to 2 months after the final dose. Infants who are HBsAg positive are considered HBV infected and should receive appropriate follow-up with a specialist.

Breastfeeding by HBV-positive mothers is considered safe and a low risk for transmission, especially if immunoprophylaxis was appropriately administered at birth. There are few data about excretion of antiviral therapies into breast milk. Complete prescribing information for all anti-HBV antivirals recommends that mothers refrain from breastfeeding while on therapy or, if breastfeeding, to discontinue antiviral use.

SUMMARY

Providing appropriate treatment and follow-up to HBV-infected mothers and their newborns is critical in preventing HBV MTCT and eradicating HBV infection. CDC guidelines recommend that all pregnant women be tested for HBsAg during each pregnancy and administration of standard passive-active immunoprophylaxis to all newborns of HBsAg-positive mothers. Although highly effective in preventing MTCT, standard passive-active immunoprophylaxis with HBIg and the hepatitis B vaccine may have a failure rate as high as 10% to 15%. Failure of immunoprophylaxis has been associated with high maternal HBV DNA levels. Hence, health care providers must consider the maternal HBV DNA level in decision making regarding management options during pregnancy. When deemed necessary, antiviral treatment can be used during pregnancy and may decrease MTCT, based on limited data. Currently, lamivudine and tenofovir remain the antiviral treatments of choice among the nucleos(t)ides for use during pregnancy. Several issues must be addressed in future clinical studies before universal recommendations for antiviral therapy for pregnant women can be made. If antiviral therapy is initiated, close monitoring during pregnancy and after delivery is necessary.

REFERENCES

1. Gambarin-Gelwan M. Hepatitis B in pregnancy. Clin Liver Dis 2007;11(4):945–63.
2. Alter MJ. Epidemiology of hepatitis B in Europe and worldwide. J Hepatol 2003; 39(Suppl 1):S64–9.
3. Tran T. Hepatitis B and pregnancy. Curr Hepat Rep 2009;8(4):154–6.
4. Jonas M. Hepatitis B and pregnancy: an underestimated issue. Liver Int 2009; 29(Suppl 1):133–9.
5. Gupta I, Ratho RK. Immunogenicity and safety of two schedules of Hepatitis B vaccination during pregnancy. J Obstet Gynaecol Res 2003;29(2):84–6.
6. Tran TT, Keeffe EB. Management of the pregnant hepatitis B patient. Curr Hepat Rep 2008;2:43–8.

7. World Health Organization. Hepatitis B. World Health Organization fact sheet 204. Available at: http://who.int/inf-fs/en/fact204.html. Accessed November 2009.
8. Centers for Disease Control and Prevention. Implementation of newborn hepatitis B vaccination—worldwide, 2006. MMWR Morb Mortal Wkly Rep 2008;57(46): 1249–52.
9. del Canho R, Grosheide PM, Schalm SW, et al. Failure of neonatal hepatitis B vaccination: the role of HBV-DNA levels in hepatitis B carrier mothers and HLA antigens in neonates. J Hepatol 1994;20(4):483–6.
10. Wiseman E, Fraser MA, Holden S, et al. Perinatal transmission of hepatitis B virus: an Australian experience. Med J Aust 2009;190:489–92.
11. Ngui SL, O'Connell S, Eglin RP, et al. Low detection rate and maternal provenance of hepatitis B virus S gene mutants in cases of failed postnatal immunoprophylaxis in England and Wales. J Infect Dis 1997;176(5):1360–5.
12. Lee SD, Lo KJ, Tsai YT, et al. Maternal hepatitis B virus DNA in mother infant transmission. Lancet 1989;1(8640):719.
13. Karthigesu VD, Allison LM, Ferguson M, et al. A hepatitis B virus variant found in the sera of immunised children induces a conformational change in the HBsAg "a" determinant. J Med Virol 1999;58(4):346–52.
14. US Food and Drug Administration. Code of federal regulations. Title 21. Volume 4, Part 201-Labeling. Revised April 2009. Available at: http://www.accessdata.fda. gov/scripts/cdrh/cfdocs/cfcfr/cfrsearch.cfm?fr=201.57. Accessed November 28, 2009.
15. European Association for the Study of the Liver. EASL clinical practice guidelines: management of chronic hepatitis B. J Hepatol 2009;50:227–42.
16. Lok AS, McMahon BJ, Practice Guideline Committee, American Association for the Study of Liver Disease, AASLD Practice Guidelines. Chronic Hepatitis B: Update 2009. Hepatology 2009;50(3):661–2.
17. Keeffe EB, Dieterich DT, Han SB, et al. A treatment algorithm for the management of chronic hepatitis B virus infection in the United States: 2008 update. Clin Gastroenterol Hepatol 2008;6(12):1315–41 [quiz: 1286].
18. Fontana RJ. Side effects of long-term oral antiviral therapy for hepatitis B. Hepatology 2009;49(Suppl 5):S185–95.
19. U.S. Preventive Services Task Force. Screening for hepatitis B virus infection in pregnancy: U.S. Preventive Services Task Force reaffirmation recommendation statement. Ann Intern Med 2009;150(12):869–73 W154.
20. Weinbaum CM, Williams I, Mast EE, et al. Recommendations for identification and public health management of persons with chronic hepatitis B virus infection. MMWR Recomm Rep 2008;57:1–20.
21. ACOG Committee on Practice Bulletins-Gynecology. ACOG Practice Bulletin No. 86: viral hepatitis in pregnancy. Obstet Gynecol 2007;110:941–55.
22. Ornoy A, Tenebaum A. Pregnancy outcome following infections by coxsackie, echo, measles, mumps, hepatitis, polio, and encephalitis virus. Reprod Toxicol 2006;21:446–57.
23. Liaw YF, Leung N, Kao JH, et al. Asian-Pacific consensus statement on the management of chronic hepatitis B: a 2008 update. Hepatol Int 2008;2: 263–83.
24. Xu D, Yan Y, Choi BC, et al. Risk factors and mechanism of transplacental transmission of hepatitis B virus: a case-control study. J Med Virol 2002;67(1):20–6.
25. Lin HH, Lee TY, Chen DS, et al. Transplacental leakage of HBeAg-positive maternal blood as the most likely route in causing intrauterine infection with hepatitis B virus. J Pediatr 1987;111:877–81.

26. Burk RD, Hwang LY, Ho GY, et al. Outcome of perinatal hepatitis B virus exposure is dependent on maternal virus load. J Infect Dis 1994;170:1418–23.
27. Pande C, Kumar A, Patra S, et al. High maternal hepatitis virus DNA levels but not HBeAg positivity predicts perinatal transmission of hepatitis B to the newborn. Gastroenterology 2008;134:A-760.
28. Su G, Pan K, Zhao N, et al. Efficacy and safety of lamivudine treatment for chronic hepatitis B in pregnancy. World J Gastroenterol 2004;10(6):910–2.
29. Tang JR, Hsu HY, Lin HH, et al. Hepatitis B surface antigenemia at birth: a long-term follow-up study. J Pediatr 1998;133(3):374–7.
30. del Canho R, Grosheide PM, Mazel JA, et al. Ten-year neonatal hepatitis B vaccination program, The Netherlands, 1982–1992: protective efficacy and long-term immunogenicity. Vaccine 1997;15(15):1624–30.
31. Ip HM, Lelie PN, Wong VC, et al. Prevention of hepatitis B virus carrier state in infants according to maternal serum levels of HBV DNA. Lancet 1989;1(8635):406–10.
32. Connor EM, Sperling RS, Gelber R, et al. Reduction of maternal-infant transmission of human immunodeficiency virus type 1 with zidovudine treatment. Pediatric AIDS Clinical Trials Group Protocol 076 Study Group. N Engl J Med 1994;331(18): 1173–80.
33. Antiretroviral Pregnancy Registry Steering Committee. Antiretroviral pregnancy registry international interim report for 1 January 1989 through 31 January 2009. Wilmington (NC): Registry Coordinating Center; 2009. Available at: http://www.APRegistry.com. Accessed November 26, 2009.
34. Dybul M, Fauci AS, Bartlett JG, et al. Guidelines for using antiretroviral agents among HIV-infected adults and adolescents. Recommendations on the Panel on Clinical Practices for the Treatment of HIV. MMWR Recomm Rep 2002;51: 1–55.
35. Bridges EG, Selden JR, Luo S. Nonclinical safety profile of telbivudine, a novel potent antiviral agent for treatment of hepatitis B. Antimicrob Agents Chemother 2008;52(7):2521–8.
36. Peters MG. Special populations with hepatitis B virus infection. Hepatology 2009; 49(5 Suppl):S146.
37. Lok AS, Fleischer R, Liang TJ, et al. Management of hepatitis B: summary of a clinical research workshop. Hepatology 2007;45(4):1056–75.
38. Tyrell DJL, Mitchell MC, De Man RA, et al. Phase II trial of lamivudine for chronic hepatitis B. Hepatology 1993;18:112 (A).
39. Mirochnick M, Capparelli E. Pharmacokinetics of antiretrovirals in pregnant women. Clin Pharmacokinet 2004;43(15):1071–87.
40. Johnson MA, Moore KH, Yuen GJ, et al. Clinical pharmacokinetics of lamivudine. Clin Pharmacokinet 1999;36(1):41–66.
41. van Zonneveld M, van Nunen AB, Niesters HG, et al. Lamivudine treatment during pregnancy to prevent perinatal transmission of hepatitis B virus infection. J Viral Hepat 2003;10(4):294–7.
42. Xu WM, Cui YT, Wang L, et al. Lamivudine in late pregnancy to prevent perinatal transmission of hepatitis B virus infection: a multicentre, randomized, double-blind, placebo-controlled study. J Viral Hepat 2009;16(2):94–103.
43. Chotiyaputta W, Lok AS. Role of antiviral therapy in the prevention of perinatal transmission of hepatitis B virus infection [editorial]. J Viral Hepat 2009;16:91–3.
44. Dienstag JL, Schiff ER, Wright TL, et al. Lamivudine as initial treatment for chronic hepatitis B in the United States. N Engl J Med 1999;341(17):1256–63.
45. ter Borg MJ, Leemans WF, de Man RA, et al. Exacerbation of chronic hepatitis B infection after delivery. J Viral Hepat 2008;15(1):37–41.

46. Tran T. Management of hepatitis B in pregnancy: weighing the options. Cleve Clin J Med 2009;76(Suppl 3):S25–9.

47. Fwu C-W, Chien Y-C, Kirk GD, et al. Hepatitis B virus infection and hepatocellular carcinoma among parous Taiwanese women: nationwide cohort study. J Natl Cancer Inst 2009;101:1019–72.

48. Mast EE, Margolis HS, Fiore, et al. A comprehensive immunization strategy to eliminate transmission of hepatitis B virus infection in the United States: recommendations of the Advisory Committee on Immunization Practices (ACIP) part 1: immunization of infants, children, and adolescents. MMWR Recomm Rep 2005;54:1–31.

Management of Hepatitis B in Special Patient Populations

Hank S. Wang, MD, Steven-Huy B. Han, MD, AGAF*

KEYWORDS

- Acute liver failure • Hepatitis B and C coinfection
- Hepatitis B and HIV coinfection
- Immunosuppression-associated hepatitis B reactivation

Acute liver failure (ALF) is characterized by coagulopathy and encephalopathy in a patient without preexisting cirrhosis.[1] In the United States and the United Kingdom, acetaminophen toxicity remains the leading cause of ALF, while acute hepatitis B virus (HBV) infection makes up approximately 7% to 19% of all cases.[2] In contrast, in Asia, HBV is a more common cause of ALF, accounting for 21% to 38% of all cases based on studies from different countries.[3] The clinical spectrum of acute HBV infection varies from subclinical, asymptomatic hepatitis to fulminant hepatic failure.

Patients with ALF secondary to acute HBV who do not undergo liver transplantation (LT) have, in general, a poor prognosis, with a published survival rate between 19% to 33%.[4] These individuals have a worse overall prognosis than ALF secondary to other etiologies.[2] LT is the only therapeutic treatment shown to prevent death, and it is associated with a greater than 80% survival in ALF caused by acute HBV.[5] LT, however, is limited by availability of donor organs and by high rates of HBV recurrence (estimated to be 20%) following LT.[5]

No randomized controlled trials have been performed evaluating the efficacy of medical treatment in patients with ALF caused by acute HBV. Existing studies in acute HBV infection, however, suggest that there may be a benefit in initiating antiviral therapy in patients with ALF caused by HBV. Just as importantly, nucleoside analog antiviral therapy is safe and well tolerated in chronic HBV[6] and in decompensated liver disease.[7] Furthermore, antiviral therapy reduces the risk of HBV recurrence following LT. Medical therapy with interferon, in contrast, may accelerate existing liver disease in ALF[8] and is not recommended for use in the acute disease setting.

Three major studies have been performed to date looking at the role of medical therapy in ALF due to HBV. In 2004, Schmilovitz-Weiss and colleagues[9] published

Division of Digestive Diseases, Dumont-UCLA Liver Transplant Center, David Geffen School of Medicine at University of California Los Angeles, Los Angeles, CA 90095, USA
* Corresponding author. Pfleger Liver Institute, 200 UCLA Medical Plaza, Suite 214, Los Angeles, CA 90095.
E-mail address: steven.han@ucla.edu

Clin Liver Dis 14 (2010) 505–520
doi:10.1016/j.cld.2010.05.002
1089-3261/10/$ – see front matter. Published by Elsevier Inc.

liver.theclinics.com

a prospective pilot study evaluating the use of lamivudine treatment (100 mg daily for 3 to 6 months) in 15 patients with severe acute HBV (defined by the presence of two of the following criteria: hepatic encephalopathy, serum bilirubin $\geq$ 10.0 mg/dL, or international normalized ratio [INR] $\geq$ 1.6). Thirteen patients (86.7%) responded to treatment with resolution of hepatic encephalopathy within 3 days and coagulopathy within 1 week. Two patients who received delayed therapy by 6 weeks developed fulminant hepatitis requiring urgent LT. In responders, serum HBV DNA was undetectable within 4 weeks, and serum liver enzymes normalized within 8 weeks. All patients tolerated lamivudine without any reported adverse events.

In 2006, Tillman and colleagues[10] evaluated lamivudine therapy (either 100 or 150 mg daily) in patients with acute (INR >2.0) or fulminant (hepatic encephalopathy) HBV and found that 14 of 17 (82.4%) lamivudine-treated patients survived without LT. Twelve of these patients had normalization of prothrombin time and a decrease in total bilirubin within a week of therapy, while all 14 cleared hepatitis B surface antigen (HBsAg) within 6 months of therapy. The three nonresponders included patients with the most severe liver disease (as indicated by severe coagulopathy) or concomitant acetaminophen ingestion (>5 g). The authors compared this series with a historic control of 20 patients, wherein only 4 patients not receiving lamivudine survived without LT. No drug-related adverse events were recorded.

Finally, a randomized controlled trial comparing lamivudine 100 mg daily for 3 months versus placebo in the treatment of acute HBV found no difference in clinical or biochemical improvement between the two groups. The study included all patients with acute HBV. Severe acute viral hepatitis was defined by the presence of two of three criteria: hepatic encephalopathy, serum bilirubin greater than or equal to 10.0 mg/dL, or INR greater than or equal to 1.6. Only 22 of 31 patients in the lamivudine treatment group and 25 of 40 patients in the placebo group met the definition for severe acute viral hepatitis. Only two patients in the lamivudine group and one in the placebo group had hepatic encephalopathy. Overall, no differences in HBV DNA, serum bilirubin, alanine aminotransferase (ALT), and INR were seen up to 1 year after treatment between the two groups.[11]

A retrospective study by the Acute Liver Failure Study Group (ALFSG) reported as an abstract evaluated whether use of nucleoside analogs favorably influenced outcomes in ALF caused by HBV. Of 57 patients with HBV ALF, 32 (56.1%) received a nucleoside analog (29 lamivudine, 1 adefovir/lamivudine, and 2 entecavir), with a median duration of therapy for 9 days (range 1 to 36 days). The treatment group that received a nucleoside analog was significantly older (51 vs 38 years), had significantly greater bilirubin levels (23.4 mg/dL vs 15.2 mg/dL), and had lower ALT (1234 IU/L vs 2416 IU/L) and significantly lower aspartate aminotransferase (AST) levels (676 IU/L vs 1347 IU/L). Overall survival was similar. The authors concluded that no benefit for antiviral therapy was identified in ALF caused by HBV, although selection bias and differences in treatment duration likely confounded reported results.[12]

Wai and colleagues[13] evaluated clinical features and prognostic factors in patients with ALF caused by HBV and found that advanced age was the only independent factor associated with a poor outcome, while no laboratory test predicted outcome. Although virologic factors have not been shown to affect overall survival in patients with ALF caused by acute HBV, some viral factors may be important in determining who develops ALF. Specifically, the presence of precore stop codon ($G_{1896}A$) and core promoter dual ($T_{1762}A$, $A_{1764}T$) variants is associated with an increased risk for development of ALF caused by HBV.[13] HBV genotype D also has been found to have a greater association with ALF caused by HBV, suggesting that this genotype may be associated with a more aggressive disease course. Overall, given the potential benefit of antiviral therapy in patients with ALF caused by acute HBV weighed against minimal risks of therapy, most would recommend initiating antiviral therapy in ALF caused by HBV.

HEPATITIS B AND C COINFECTION

The exact worldwide prevalence of hepatitis C virus (HCV) coinfection with HBV is unknown due in part to the unknown prevalence of occult HBV infection. Some have estimated the prevalence of HCV coinfection to range between 7% and 15% of all patients with chronic HBV infection.[14] Patients with combined HBV and HCV coinfection exhibit a spectrum of virologic profiles, as levels of viremia appear to vary over time due to viral interference between hepatotropic viruses. Clinically, HCV inhibition of HBV replication is more commonly seen than the reverse. In vitro studies suggest that HCV suppression of HBV replication may be mediated by HCV core protein[15] and may be genotype-dependent.[16] In contrast, some other studies have suggested either a reciprocal interference or an even greater interference by HBV on HCV replication.[17] Finally, an Italian multicenter longitudinal study followed 133 untreated HBV and HCV coinfected patients for up to 1 year and found that virologic patterns in coinfected individuals are widely divergent and dynamic, with 31% demonstrating fluctuating HBV or HCV viremia levels at different time points, suggesting that HBV and HCV may alternate their dominance over different periods of coinfection.[18]

Coinfection is associated with more severe liver disease as compared with monoinfection with either HBV or HCV alone. Zarski and colleagues[19] reported more severe histologic lesions in coinfected patients, including greater prevalence of cirrhosis, piecemeal necrosis, and fibrosis as compared with HCV monoinfection. Similarly, in the previously described multicenter Italian study, cirrhosis was seen in 15.1% of HBV monoinfected patients as compared with 28.8% of coinfected patients.[20] In addition, coinfection has been shown in several studies to carry a consistent increased risk of hepatocellular carcinoma (HCC).[21] In another Italian study of cirrhotics followed longitudinally (average follow-up 64.5 months), 40% of coinfected patients compared with 20% of HCV monoinfected patients and 9% of HBV monoinfected patients developed HCC.[22]

Although no formal treatment guidelines exist, most recommend treatment targeting the dominant virus in coinfected patients.[23] Interferon has been the most widely studied therapy in coinfected patients given its known activity against both HBV and HCV. Several Taiwanese studies have evaluated combination therapy with interferon and ribavirin at various doses in coinfected patients, reporting virologic suppression rates for HBV ranging between 11% and 35.5% and sustained virologic response (SVR) rates for HCV ranging between 43% and 69%. No significant difference in SVR for HCV was seen between coinfected patients and HCV monoinfected patients (range 60% to 71%).[24–26] Recently, treatment with peginterferon alfa-2a and ribavirin was evaluated in 321 Taiwanese patients with active HCV infection, half of whom were also HBsAg positive. In HCV genotype 1, at 24 weeks after treatment (peginterferon alfa-2a 180 µg weekly for 48 weeks and ribavirin 1000 to 1200 mg daily), similar rates of SVR were reported in the monoinfected group as in the coinfected group (SVR 72.2% in coinfected patients vs 77.3% in monoinfected). At 24 weeks after treatment in HCV genotype 2 (peginterferon alfa-2a weekly for 24 weeks and ribavirin 800 mg daily), the SVR was 82.8% in coinfected and 84.0% in monoinfected patients. Overall, post-treatment HBsAg clearance was reported in 11.2% of dual-infected patients.[27]

Treatment of active HBV and HCV coinfection with interferon and lamivudine has been evaluated in only one study.[28] Eight patients were treated with 5 million units interferon and 100 mg/day lamivudine for 12 months followed by lamivudine alone for an additional 6 months. Following therapy, HCV SVR was 50%, Hepatitis B e antigen (HBe) Ag clearance was seen in three patients (two seroconverted to anti-HBe), and three patients had clearance of HBV DNA by polymerase chain reaction (PCR), although in two patients HBV DNA became detectable again by the end of the follow-up period. Given the possibility that HCV coinfection might affect response to HBV treatment, some recommend treatment of HCV first before a long-term course of nucleoside analog therapy is initiated.

HEPATITIS B AND D COINFECTION

Its been estimated that 5% of HBV carriers worldwide are coinfected with hepatitis D (delta) virus (HDV),[14] a defective virus that requires the presence of HBV to express virulence. The greatest prevalence of HDV coinfection has been described in the Mediterranean Basin, South America, and parts of Asia. Chronic HDV infection is less common in the United States and Northern Europe, where it is thought to affect only 1% of HBV-infected individuals.

Coinfection with HDV is associated with more severe liver disease and a greater incidence of cirrhosis than HBV monoinfection. Specifically, in Asia, where the predominant genotype is genotype 2, a less severe course has been reported with coinfection with HDV than with HCV. Liaw and colleagues[29] followed individuals with HBV coinfected with acute HCV or acute HDV for up to 20 years and found an overall mortality of 10% in HCV coinfected patients and 7% in HDV coinfected patients, with cirrhosis seen in 48% of HCV coinfected and in 21% of HDV coinfected patients. In contrast, in the West, where genotype 1 predominates, a more severe course has been described in HDV coinfection. A prospective Italian study looked at over 800 patients with HBsAg positivity and found that cirrhosis was present in 107 of the 709 patients (15.1%) with HBV alone, in 30 of 69 patients (43%) with hepatitis D virus coinfection, and in 17 of 59 patients (28.8%) with HCV coinfection.[20]

The primary goal of therapy lies in suppressing HDV replication, which usually is associated with normalization of serum aminotransferases and improvement in inflammatory grade on liver biopsy. Interferon alfa, the only drug currently approved for treatment of chronic HDV, has shown mixed results in various studies. In one case report, long-term therapy with interferon alfa at high doses (5 million units daily for 12 years) led to resolution of chronic HDV, disappearance of HDV and HBV markers, and improvement in fibrosis.[30] In the largest multicenter trial published to date, 61 Italian patients with chronic HDV were randomly assigned to either interferon alfa (three times a week at 5 million units/m2 for 4 months followed by three times a week at 3 million units/m2 for another 8 months) or no treatment and were followed for 12 additional months following the end of therapy. Overall, histologic improvement (57% of treated vs 36% of untreated patients) and suppression of HDV replication (45% of treated vs 27% of controls) was similar between the two groups suggesting a lack of benefit with short-term therapy.[31]

In a smaller study, 36 patients with chronic HDV were randomized to a 48-week course of high-dose (9 million units) or low dose (3 million units) interferon alfa or no treatment and were followed for an additional 2 to 14 years. Survival was significantly greater in the high dose group compared with the low-dose group and controls; no survival benefit was seen with low-dose treatment when compared with controls. Furthermore, patients in the high-dose group had improved liver histology (improved inflammation and fibrosis) and were more likely to have clearance of HDV RNA and HBV DNA as compared with those in the other groups.[32]

There are a limited number of studies evaluating the role of pegylated interferon in the treatment of chronic HDV.[33–36] Recently, 12 patients with chronic HDV were prospectively treated with 1.5 μg/kg peginterferon-alfa-2b for 48 weeks and then followed for 24 weeks. A sustained response (undetectable HDV RNA and normalization of ALT at 6 months after treatment) was seen in only 2 of 12 patients (17%). However, nonresponders were identified by a less than 3 log decrease of HDV RNA at 6 months of therapy (negative predictive value 100%). Histologic scores improved in responders compared with nonresponders at the end of follow-up.[33]

The largest published study looked at 38 patients treated with peginterferon-alfa-2b (1.5 μg/kg) alone as monotherapy or in combination with ribavirin for 48 weeks. Thereafter, all patients received peginterferon for 24 weeks and were followed for 24 weeks off therapy. The overall response rate in terms of virologic response (19% monotherapy vs 9% combination therapy) and biochemical response (37.5% monotherapy vs 41% combination therapy) was similar, suggesting no additional benefit of ribavirin on viral clearance. More patients on combination therapy (63%) had to undergo dose modification compared with those on monotherapy (50%).[34] Finally, few studies have evaluated combination therapy for HDV using interferon with nucleoside analogs, but the available data suggest little increased effect on HDV infection, serum aminotransferase levels, or histology compared with interferon monotherapy alone.[37,38]

HBV AND HUMAN IMMUNODEFICIENCY VIRUS COINFECTION

Human immunodeficiency virus-1 (HIV) and HBV share common modes of transmission through sexual and percutaneous routes, making coinfection with both viruses unsurprisingly common. Worldwide coinfection prevalence depends largely on HBV endemicity. In countries with low HBV endemicity, including the United States and Europe, the prevalence of HBV coinfection is thought to range between 5% and 7% of the HIV-infected population[39]; in countries with greater HBV endemicity, due primarily to vertical transmission, HBV infection can precede HIV infection by decades, and the overall prevalence of coinfection can be up to 10% to 20% of all HIV-infected individuals.[40]

The success of highly active antiretroviral therapy (HAART) in the United States and other industrialized countries has reduced deaths from acquired immunodeficiency syndrome (AIDS)-related causes. As a result, HIV-infected patients are living longer, and liver-related disease, along with heart disease, has become one of the leading causes of morbidity and mortality in these patients. With regard to HBV, HIV infection exacerbates every phase of the natural history of adult-acquired HBV. HIV patients have

Up to a sixfold increased risk of developing chronic hepatitis B after acute infection[41]

Up to a fivefold decreased likelihood of HBe clearance[42]

Increased levels of HBV replication as evidenced by higher serum HBV DNA levels[43]

A greater chance for loss of hepatitis B surface antibody (anti-HBs) and subsequent reactivation of HBV.[44]

Furthermore, HIV increases the rate of HBV-related liver disease, including cirrhosis and HBV-related mortality. Thio and colleagues[45] found that HIV-HBV coinfected patients were nearly 20 times more likely to die of liver-related illness compared with HBV monoinfected patients.

Several serologic phenomena are seen in individuals with HIV and HBV coinfection. Coinfected patients may undergo spontaneous reverse seroconversion, characterized by loss of anti-HBs and recurrence of HBsAg particularly in the presence of low CD4 counts (<200 cells/mm^3), which leads to an increased risk of HBV reactivation.[44] In addition, an isolated hepatitis B core antigen antibody (anti-HBc) serologic pattern is seen in many coinfected individuals, which is of unclear clinical significance as no clear liver disease has been found to be associated with presence of anti-HBc.[46] The presence of anti-HBc alone can signify exposure with subsequent loss of anti-HBs, occult HBV infection, or a false-positive test result. In coinfected patients with anti-HBc, the presence of latent hepatitis B, marked by the presence of HBV DNA, ranged from a few percent up to 89% in one study of patients followed serially.[47]

Indications for treatment of HBV in HIV-infected patients are similar to those in patients with HBV monoinfection. Current guidelines recommend evaluating both the replication status of HBV along with the stage of liver disease together to determine treatment decisions. Although no definitive cutoff value has been well established, many experts recommend initiating therapy in coinfected patients at an HBV DNA level of 2000 IU/mL (approximately 10,000 copies/mL).[48] Similarly, the presence of even mild-to-moderate liver disease is an indication to initiate treatment in coinfected patients given their increased risk of fibrosis. Treatment is recommended in cirrhotics regardless of the HBV DNA level. In general, liver disease is best assessed by a liver biopsy, as aminotransferases may fluctuate in coinfected patients due to immune reconstitution or as a result of HAART-associated hepatotoxicity. Furthermore, significant liver disease may be present even in patients with normal aminotransferases, especially in those with low CD4 counts.[49]

The primary goals of therapy center on preventing disease progression, including development of cirrhosis and HCC, and reducing HBV-related morbidity and mortality. Other goals of therapy include decreasing viral replication (suppression of serum HBV DNA), HBeAg seroconversion, loss of HBsAg, and acquisition of anti-HBs, all of which are associated with improved survival and decreased incidence of HCC in HBV-monoinfected individuals.[50] Additional goals of therapy include decreasing the risk of HBV transmission to others, improving tolerability of HAART, and minimizing the risk of hepatotoxicity related to the immune reconstitution inflammatory syndrome.

Although there are no randomized controlled trials to support combination therapy in HIV coinfected patients, most specialists recommend combination therapy with two agents active against HBV to reduce the risk of HBV drug resistance. In patients who are candidates for HAART therapy (who are not yet on therapy), many recommend initial therapy with tenofovir and emtricitabine as part of an anti-HIV regimen, especially given its ease of administration and tolerability.[49] Combination therapy with medications without overlapping resistance profiles may delay onset of HBV-related drug resistance mutations.

In patients on HAART who require HBV treatment, use of a nucleoside/nucleotide analog combination (either emtricitabine and tenofovir or lamivudine and tenofovir) can be considered as long as the HIV provider is certain that there are no pre-existing HIV mutations conferring resistance to lamivudine, emtricitabine, or tenofovir. If tenofovir cannot be employed, other options include entecavir, adefovir dipivoxil, or peginterferon. In patients with complete HIV suppression who do not demonstrate YMDD motif (M204V/I) mutations in the HBV polymerase, entecavir may be the next best option given its potency and high resistance profile in both patients naïve to lamivudine therapy and patients on a lamivudine-containing regimen. Recently, however, an HIV-associated mutation, M184V, has been reported in patients on entecavir monotherapy who were treatment-naïve[51] and who previously had been treated with lamivudine.[52] Furthermore, with entecavir, there is a continued theoretical concern for increased entecavir resistance in patients on a lamivudine-containing HAART regimen given overlapping resistance patterns. In patients on a fixed HAART regimen due either to patient preference or HIV drug resistance patterns, addition of adefovir or pegylated interferon may be considered. Adefovir is active against both lamivudine-sensitive and lamivudine resistant HBV but is less potent than tenofovir. Peginterferon has not been studied in HIV-infected patients, although its safety has been demonstrated in patients with HIV/HCV.[53]

Therapy for coinfected patients who do not require HIV treatment is limited given dual activity of many nucleoside analogs and concern for development of HIV drug resistance. Currently, in addition to lamivudine, entecavir, and tenofovir, only adefovir, peginterferon-alfa, and telbivudine are available as monotherapeutic agents; while combination therapy with one or more may be effective in this scenario, it has not been studied to date. Telbivudine, the most potent of the three, is limited by concern for drug-resistant HBV seen in the monoinfected patient.[49] In contrast, with peginterferon-alfa, there is no concern for either HBV or HIV drug-resistance; however, adverse effects limit overall tolerability. Adefovir at a suboptimal concentration for HIV-1 does not appear to select for adefovir mutations at codons 65 and 70 or any other particular HIV-1 reverse transcriptase resistance profile in coinfected patients[54]; predisposition for HIV-related tenofovir resistance, however, is unknown. Alternatively, many guidelines, including the International AIDS Society-USA, are now recommending earlier initiation of HAART given concern for more severe liver disease in coinfected patients.[55] Finally, given concern for immune reconstitution inflammatory syndrome, usually seen within 4 to 8 weeks of starting HAART therapy, some experts have recommended that anti-HBV therapy be initiated before HAART therapy, especially in the presence of elevated HBV DNA levels.

IMMUNOSUPPRESSION-ASSOCIATED HEPATITIS B REACTIVATION

HBV reactivation is characterized by the reappearance of HBV DNA in a patient with prior evidence of resolved or inactive HBV infection. The clinical presentation of disease can be varied, ranging from a subclinical, asymptomatic course to severe acute hepatitis and even fulminant liver failure. Although HBV reactivation can occur spontaneously, most often it results following withdrawal of chemotherapy or immunosuppression. Reactivation is marked by three phases, including an acute increase in HBV replication that usually occurs following initiation of immunosuppression, hepatic injury that is characterized by an acute increase in serum aminotransferase levels, and ultimately recovery, whereby elevated transaminases normalize and HBV markers return to baseline levels.[56]

The exact risk of reactivation has not been well-defined and is thought to range anywhere between 20% and 50% based on several studies.[57,58] In 78 HBsAg-positive patients receiving cancer chemotherapy for various solid organ tumors excluding HCC, 19% of cases of acute hepatitis were attributed to HBV reactivation in one series.[57] In contrast, Lok and colleagues[58] found that reactivation among 27 HBsAg-positive patients with lymphoma undergoing cancer chemotherapy was 48%; furthermore, reactivation was associated with the development of jaundice in 22% of patients. Finally, a large meta-analysis analyzing 13 studies with a combined 424 patients found an overall HBV reactivation rate of 50% (range 24% to 88%).[59] Known risk factors of HBV reactivation have been described to include prechemotherapy HBV DNA level, concomitant use of steroids, and a diagnosis of lymphoma or breast cancer.[60]

Immunosuppression promotes HBV reactivation by limiting the host immune response to the virus and facilitating viral replication. Furthermore, several commonly used immunosuppressives including prednisone and azathioprine may enhance viral replication via additional direct mechanisms. In vitro corticosteroid use has been shown to increase HBV DNA and RNA synthesis via the presence of a glucocorticoid receptor binding sequence that augments glucocorticoid-dependent activity of the HBV enhancer.[61] At higher doses, azathioprine increases intracellular viral DNA and RNA levels approximately fourfold, while a combination of prednisone, azathioprine, and cyclosporine A increases the level of intracellular viral DNA eightfold, suggesting an additive effect with cyclosporine A in DNA-transfected hepatoma cells.[62] Ultimately, as immunosuppression is decreased and the host immune function is restored, rapid destruction of infected hepatocytes can lead to clinical hepatitis with a spectrum of disease presentations.

The relationship between the intensity and duration of chemotherapy or immunosuppression and the risk of HBV reactivation in patients with occult HBV infection (HBsAg negative, but HBcAb positive) has not been well described. Recently, several case reports have described severe hepatitis flares associated with rituximab, a monoclonal antibody against CD20, used to treat non-Hodgkin lymphoma. In 12 case reports of HBV reactivation due to rituximab therapy, the overall mortality rate was 83%, with 5 documented cases of reverse seroconversion or reactivation in 5 patients who were HBsAg-negative before therapy.[56] In a recent trial, 46 patients who were HBsAg negative and anti-HBc positive were treated with cyclophosphamide, doxorubicin, vincristine, and prednisone (CHOP) either with (n = 21) or without (n = 25) rituximab. In the R-CHOP group, five patients developed HBV reactivation, including one patient who died of hepatic failure; in contrast, none of the 25 patients treated with CHOP alone developed HBV reactivation. Predictive risk factors for HBV reactivation included male gender, absence of anti-HBs, and use of rituximab.[63]

Finally, HBV reactivation has been described in the setting of infliximab use. The rate of HBV reactivation and the severity of reactivation in patients receiving antitumor necrosis factor (TNF) therapy have not been well described. Furthermore, it is unclear whether all TNF-alpha antagonists confer the same risk of reactivation. The largest study evaluated HBV reactivation in 80 patients with Crohn disease with HBV markers prospectively determined before infliximab infusion. Three Crohn disease patients with chronic HBV infection were identified; two of these three developed severe reactivation of HBV following withdrawal of therapy, and one died. A third patient, who was treated with lamivudine at the onset of infliximab therapy, had no evidence of HBV reactivation.[64] In addition to this study, more than a dozen documented cases of severe HBV reactivation following the use of infliximab leading to three fatalities[56] have been reported in the literature.

Several studies have described significantly fewer cases of HBV reactivation during chemotherapy when lamivudine is given preventively. A meta-analysis of 14 studies (including 2 randomized controlled trials) found that with prophylactic lamivudine, the relative risk for both HBV reactivation and HBV-related hepatitis ranged from 0.00 to 0.21 (reduced risk by 79% to 100%) in patients undergoing chemotherapy.[59] In another study, 30 consecutive patients with lymphoma undergoing chemotherapy were randomized to lamivudine 100 mg daily 1 week before chemotherapy or to deferred treatment until serologic evidence of HBV reactivation appeared. There were no cases of HBV reactivation in the former group compared with eight (53%) cases of reactivation in the latter; furthermore, hepatitis-free survival was significantly longer in the group that received prophylactic therapy.[65] Finally, in a last study, 65 HBsAg-positive patients undergoing chemotherapy received prophylactic lamivudine for 1 week before receiving chemotherapy. These patients were compared with 193 well-matched historical HBsAg-positive controls. In the prophylactic lamivudine group, there was significantly less HBV reactivation (4.6% vs 24.4%), fewer overall cases of hepatitis (17.5% vs 44.6%), fewer severe cases of hepatitis (4.8% vs 18.7%), and less disruption of chemotherapy (15.4% vs 34.6%) as compared with the control group.[66]

HEPATITIS B IN KIDNEY AND HEART TRANSPLANT PATIENTS

In organ transplant recipients, including renal and heart transplantation, recurrent HBV most often results from HBV reactivation and not from de novo infection (either from the organ donor or from infected blood products). The clinical spectrum of presentation caused by reactivation of HBV varies from an asymptomatic hepatitis to hepatic failure and death. Fibrosing cholestatic hepatitis, characterized by an extremely high mortality and histology demonstrating hepatocyte ballooning, cholestasis, and prominent expression of HBsAg in hepatocytes, has been described in HBsAg-positive patients following renal transplantation.[67] Risk factors that may predict the severity of reactivation have not been well defined. Both patients with HBsAg positivity (including precore or basic core promoter variants and core gene mutations) and those with a history of prior infection are at risk for reactivation with immunosuppression. In one study, Lau and colleagues[68] demonstrated that a high serum HBV DNA level ($>10^5$ copies/mL) was the most important risk factor for HBV reactivation in patients undergoing autologous hematopoietic cell transplantation.

The long-term outcome of patients with untreated HBV following organ transplantation is poor. Several studies in patients following kidney transplantation have suggested decreased transplant function, more severe liver disease, and even reduced long-term survival. In one study of 151 HBsAg-positive kidney transplant recipients, followed for a median of 125 months, spontaneous disappearance rates of HBsAg, HBeAg, and HBV DNA were found to be lower, while rates of cirrhosis and HCC were found to be higher than those in the general population.[69] In a retrospective study, multivariate analysis found HBsAg positivity to be associated with an increased risk of graft failure and death, although the latter was not statistically significant.[70] In a case-controlled study, renal transplant recipients with HBsAg positivity had significantly worse outcomes, including deteriorating biochemical markers, loss of HBsAg positivity, and increased overall mortality with matched HBsAg-positive patients maintained on hemodialysis.[71]

In contrast, after heart transplantation, HBV infection does not lead to immediate significant liver disease, although it may affect long-term survival. In an older French study looking at 69 patients who developed HBV infection (mostly as a result of nosocomial transmission during endomyocardial biopsy), most had mild ALT level increases, a high level of viral replication, and few severe histologic lesions, except for patients infected by precore HBV mutants. The 5-year survival rate following heart transplantation in patients with HBV was 81%, similar to that in patients without liver test abnormalities (76%).[72] In another study following 69 HBV-infected patients after heart transplantation for a mean of 105 months, 34 patients (45.9%) died during follow-up, a significant difference when compared with the control group (28.8%). Histology of 25 HBsAg-positive patients more than 5 years after infection revealed severe fibrosis or cirrhosis in 14 (56%), mild fibrosis in 9 (36%), and chronic hepatitis without fibroproliferation in 2 (8%).[73]

While interferon therapy may cause cardiac graft rejection,[74,75] lamivudine, in contrast, has been shown to be safe and effective in treating post-transplantation HBV reactivation. Furthermore, it may be a viable therapy for ALF caused by fibrosing cholestatic hepatitis B.[76] In 1996, Liu and colleagues[77] obtained approval for compassionate use of lamivudine 100 mg/d in 15 post-transplant patients (HBsAg positive) with HBV reactivation in Taiwan (9 renal transplants, 6 heart transplants, 1 lung transplant). They reported an overall survival rate of 75% (12 of 16 patients), with 4 deaths seen in patients who initiated therapy late given elevated pretreatment serum total bilirubin (≥ 3 mg/dL). Serum HBV-DNA was undetectable in the 12 survivors (median treatment 101 weeks). Three developed lamivudine resistance 36 to 60 weeks following initiation of therapy. In a small study of six HBV DNA-positive cadaveric renal transplant patients given lamivudine on a compassionate use basis, rapid disappearance of HBV DNA from the serum was seen in all patients.[78]

In another Taiwanese series looking specifically at heart transplant recipients, 10 of 14 patients treated with lamivudine salvage therapy survived with normalized ALT and undetectable HBV DNA (duration of treatment 6 to 100 months). One patient died due to end-stage cirrhosis while awaiting liver transplantation, while two patients developed YMDD mutations at 15 and 96 months of treatment.[79] Finally, a German pilot study looked at 20 heart transplant recipients with chronic HBV, 16 of whom were switched to lamivudine (from famciclovir). Long-term response to lamivudine was reported in 37.5% (6 of 16) of patients lasting for up to 7 years. Lamivudine resistance developed in 10 patients (62.5%), although 4 of these patients were successfully treated with rescue therapy after 2003 with adefovir (n = 3) and tenofovir (n = 1). Of the nine patients who died within the 8-year follow-up period, five (56%) died from liver failure, all of whom experienced lamivudine resistance and who were not treated with rescue therapy as they died before 2003.[80]

Prolonged lamivudine therapy ultimately leads to lamivudine resistance via mutations within the HBV polymerase gene (YMDD variants). Prevalence of resistance increases with duration of exposure, and in one series, resistance was reported to be 14%, 26%, and 65% after 1, 2, and 4 years of therapy respectively.[81,82] Following transplantation, resistance is thought to accelerate primarily due to concomitant immunosuppression with steroids that enhance HBV replication. Virologic relapse rates following discontinuation of lamivudine in kidney transplant recipients have been reported to be as high as 67%,[80] prompting most to continue lamivudine indefinitely in patients with HBsAg positivity.

Diagnosis of HBV reactivation can be made based on the presence of increased HBV replication (increase in serum HBV DNA) in patients with serologic evidence of chronic or past HBV infection. Management of HBV reactivation depends on the serologic status of the transplant candidate. In patients who are HBsAg positive, the timing of lamivudine therapy after transplantation is somewhat controversial, as two approaches have been employed. Salvage treatment refers to delaying lamivudine therapy until established reactivation, whereas preemptive treatment features initiation of lamivudine immediately following transplantation. Salvage therapy may not rescue those with pre-existing liver disease or those with fibrosing cholestatic hepatitis, although it will help to minimize lamivudine resistance. In contrast, preemptive therapy is thought to minimize both early and late liver-related mortality at the cost of perhaps greater lamivudine resistance. In HBsAg-positive patients, most initiate pre-emptive nucleoside analog therapy before immunosuppression, because ALT and HBV DNA levels are lowest before corticosteroid-enhanced HBV replication, which when it occurs increases the risk of post-transplant lamivudine resistance.[83]

In cases where progression to HBV-related liver failure has occurred despite lamivudine therapy, late initiation of nucleoside analog therapy has been attributed to treatment failure in those patients.[84] The appropriate time and length of therapy have not been well established, and in some select patients without evidence of active disease, discontinuation of nucleoside analog therapy has been suggested to minimize the development of drug-resistant HBV mutations.[85,86] The prevalence of YMDD HBV mutant has been shown to be 15% by week 52 and 38% by week 104 in patients on continuous lamivudine therapy.[87] All patients on lamivudine should undergo tri-monthly checks of HBV DNA and ALT with a change to monthly ALT checks if the DNA is found to rise. In patients who develop YMDD-associated flares, addition of adefovir or another nucleotide analog should be considered in combination with lamivudine.[88]

Finally, patients who are anti-HBc positive with or without anti-HBs are at increased risk for reactivation. These patients should undergo serial monitoring and testing for ALT and HBV DNA while on immunosuppression, with initiation of nucleoside/nucleotide analogs once reactivation is detected. Newer nucleoside/nucleotide analogs, including entecavir, tenofovir, and emtricitabine have not been evaluated for use in preventing reactivation in these immunosuppressed organ transplant recipients.

SUMMARY

The management of HBV infection in special populations is ever changing, driven by the emergence of newer antivirals and advances in the understanding of HBV, its role in coinfection, and its risk of reactivation following immunosuppression. In ALF caused by HBV, antiviral therapy should be initiated without delay given minimal risk of therapy. In HBV patients coinfected with HCV, treatment of HCV first generally is recommended before a long course of nucleoside analog therapy is initiated. Interferon alfa is the only drug approved for the treatment of chronic HDV infection; combination therapy with ribavirin or a nucleoside analog does not appear to enhance virologic response. In HIV coinfected patients, combination therapy with two agents active against HBV should be employed to minimize risk of HBV drug resistance. Finally, in HBsAg-positive patients, preemptive nucleoside analog therapy should be started before immunosuppression given concern for corticosteroid-enhanced HBV replication.

REFERENCES

1. Polson J, Lee WM. AASLD position paper: the management of acute liver failure. Hepatology 2005;41:1179–97.
2. Ostapowicz G, Fontana RJ, Schiodt FV, et al. Results of a prospective study of acute liver failure at 17 tertiary care centers in the United States. Ann Intern Med 2002;137:947–54.
3. Lee H. Acute liver failure related to hepatitis B virus. Hepatol Res 2008;38:S9–13.
4. Shakil AO, Kramer D, Mazariegos GV, et al. Acute liver failure: clinical features, outcome analysis, and applicability of prognostic criteria. Liver Transpl 2000;6: 163–9.
5. Steinmuller T, Seehofer D, Rayes N, et al. Increasing applicability of liver transplantation for patients with hepatitis B-related liver disease. Hepatology 2002; 35:1528–35.
6. Lai CL, Chien RN, Leung NW, et al. A one-year trial of lamivudine for chronic hepatitis B. N Engl J Med 1999;329:61–8.
7. Fontanta RJ. Management of patients with decompensated HBV cirrhosis. Semin Liver Dis 2003;23:89–100.

8. Leifeled L, Cheng S, Ramakers J, et al. Imbalanced intrahepatic expression of interleukin 12, interferon gamma, and interleukin 10 in fulminant hepatitis B. Hepatology 2002;36:1001–8.

9. Schmilovitz-Weiss H, Ben-Ari Z, Sikuler E, et al. Lamivudine treatment for acute severe hepatitis B: a pilot study. Liver Int 2004;24:547–51.

10. Tillman HL, Hadem J, Leifeld L, et al. Safety and efficacy of lamivudine in patients with severe acute or fulminant hepatitis B, a multicenter experience. J Viral Hepat 2006;13:256–63.

11. Kumar M, Satapathy S, Monga R. A randomized controlled trial of lamivudine to treat acute hepatitis B. Hepatology 2007;45:97–101.

12. Seremba E, Sanders CM, Jain MK, et al. Use of nucleoside analogues in HBV-related acute liver failure. Hepatology 2007;46:276a.

13. Wai CT, Fontana RJ, Polson J, et al. Clinical outcome and virologic characteristics of hepatitis B-related acute liver failure in the United States. J Viral Hepat 2005; 12:192–8.

14. Peters MG. Special populations with hepatitis B virus infection. Hepatology 2009; 49(Suppl 5):S146–55.

15. Shih CM, Chen CM, Chen SY, et al. Modulation of the trans-suppression activity of hepatitis C virus core protein by phosphorylation. J Virol 1995;69(2):1160–71.

16. Schüttler CG, Fiedler N, Schmidt K, et al. Suppression of hepatitis B virus enhancer 1 and 2 by hepatitis C virus core protein. J Hepatol 2002;37:855–62.

17. Pontisso P, Gerotto M, Ruvoletto MG, et al. Hepatitis C genotypes in patients with dual hepatitis B and C virus infection. J Med Virol 1996;48:157–60.

18. Raimondo G, Brunetto MR, Pontisso P, et al. Longitudinal evaluation reveals a complex spectrum of virologic profiles in hepatitis B virus/hepatitis C virus-coinfected patients. Hepatology 2006;43(1):100–7.

19. Zarski JP, Bohn B, Bastie A, et al. Characteristics of patients with dual infection by hepatitis B and C viruses. J Hepatol 1998;28:27–33.

20. Gaeta GB, Stornaiuolo G, Precone DF, et al. Epidemiological and clinical burden of chronic hepatitis B virus/hepatitis C virus infection. A multicenter Italian study. J Hepatol 2003;39(6):1036–41.

21. Kaklamani E, Trichopoulos D, Tzonou A, et al. Hepatitis B and C viruses and their interaction in the origin of hepatocellular carcinoma. JAMA 1991;265:1974–6.

22. Chiaramonte M, Stroffolini T, Vian A, et al. Rate of incidence of hepatocellular carcinoma in patients with compensated viral cirrhosis. Cancer 1999;85: 2132–7.

23. Chu CJ, Lee SD. Hepatitis B virus/hepatitis C virus coinfection: epidemiology, clinical features, viral interactions, and treatment. J Gastroenterol Hepatol 2008;23(4):512–20.

24. Liu CJ, Chen PJ, Lai MY, et al. Ribavirin and interferon is effective for hepatitis C virus clearance in hepatitis B and C dually infected patients. Hepatology 2003; 37(3):568–76.

25. Hung CH, Lee CM, Lu SN, et al. Combination therapy with interferon-alpha and ribavirin in patients with dual hepatitis B and hepatitis C virus infection. J Gastroenterol Hepatol 2005;20:727–32.

26. Chuang WL, Dai CY, Chang WY, et al. Viral interaction and responses in chronic hepatitis C and B coinfected patients with interferon-alpha plus ribavirin combination therapy. Antivir Ther 2005;10:125–33.

27. Liu CJ, Chuang WL, Lee CM, et al. Peginterferon alfa-2a plus ribavirin for the treatment of dual chronic infection with hepatitis B and C viruses. Gastroenterology 2009;136:496–504.

28. Marrone A, Zampino R, D'Onofrio M, et al. Combined interferon plus lamivudine treatment in young patients with dual HBV (HBeAg positive) and HCV chronic infection. J Hepatol 2004;41(6):1064–5.
29. Liaw YF, Chen YC, Sheen IS, et al. Impact of acute hepatitis C virus superinfection in patients with chronic hepatitis B virus infection. Gastroenterology 2004;126(4): 1024–9.
30. Lau DT, Kleiner DE, Park Y, et al. Resolution of chronic delta hepatitis after 12 years of interferon alfa therapy. Gastroenterology 1999;117(5):1229–33.
31. Rosina F, Pintus C, Meschievitz C, et al. A randomized controlled trial of a 12-month course of recombinant human interferon-alpha in chronic delta (type D) hepatitis: a multicenter Italian study. Hepatology 1991;13(6): 1052–6.
32. Farci P, Roskams T, Chessa L, et al. Long-term benefit of interferon alpha therapy of chronic hepatitis D: regression of advanced hepatic fibrosis. Gastroenterology 2004;126(7):1740–9.
33. Erhardt A, Gerlich W, Starke C, et al. Treatment of chronic hepatitis delta with pegylated interferon-alpha2b. Liver Int 2006;26(7):805–10.
34. Niro GA, Ciancio A, Gaeta GB, et al. Pegylated interferon alpha-2b as monotherapy or in combination with ribavirin in chronic hepatitis delta. Hepatology 2006;44: 713–20.
35. Castelnau C, Le Gal F, Ripault MP, et al. Efficacy of peginterferon alpha-2b in chronic hepatitis delta: Relevance of quantitative RT-PCR for follow-up. Hepatology 2006;44:728–35.
36. Ferenci P, Formann E, Romeo R. Successful treatment of chronic hepatitis D with a short course of peginterferon alfa-2a. Am J Gastroenterol 2005;100: 1626–7.
37. Yurdaydin C, Wedemeyer H, Dalekos G, et al. A multicenter randomised study comparing the efficacy of pegylated interferon alfa-2A plus adefovir dipivoxil vs. pegylated interferon alfa-2A plus placebo vs. adefovir dipovoxil for the treatment of chronic delta hepatitis: the intervention trial (HID-IT) [abstract]. Hepatology 2006;41(Suppl 1):230A.
38. Yurdaydin C, Bozkaya H, Onder FO, et al. Treatment of chronic delta hepatitis with lamivudine vs lamivudine + interferon vs interferon. J Viral Hepat 2008; 15(4):314–21.
39. Alter MJ. Epidemiology of viral hepatitis and HIV co-infection. J Hepatol 2006; 44(Suppl 1):S6–9.
40. Diop-Ndiaye H, Toure-Kane C, Etard JF, et al. Hepatitis B, C seroprevalence and delta viruses in HIV-1 Senegalese patients at HAART initiation (retrospective study). J Med Virol 2008;80:1332–6.
41. Bodsworth NJ, Cooper DA, Donovan B. The influence of human immunodeficiency virus type 1 infection on the development of the hepatitis B carrier state. J Infect Dis 1991;163:1138–40.
42. Gilson RJ, Hawkins AE, Beecham MR, et al. Interactions between HIV and hepatitis B virus in homosexual men: effects on the natural history of infection. AIDS 1997;11:597–606.
43. Colin JF, Cazals-Hatem D, Loriot MA, et al. Influence of human immunodeficiency virus infection on chronic hepatitis B in homosexual men. Hepatology 1999;29: 1306–10.
44. Biggar RJ, Goedert JJ, Hoofnagle J. Accelerated loss of antibody to hepatitis B surface antigen among immunodeficient homosexual men infected with HIV. N Engl J Med 1987;316:630.

45. Thio CL, Seaberg EC, Skolasky RL, et al. HIV-1, hepatitis B virus and risk of liver-related mortality in the Multicenter AIDS Cohort Study (MACS). Lancet 2002;360: 1921–6.
46. Grob P, Jilg W, Bornhak H, et al. Serological pattern "anti-HBc alone": report on a workshop. J Med Virol 2000;62:450–5.
47. Hofer M, Joller-Jemelka HI, Grob PJ, et al. Frequent chronic hepatitis B virus infection in HIV-infected patients positive for antibody to hepatitis B core antigen only. Swiss HIV Cohort Study. Eur J Clin Microbiol Infect Dis 1998; 17:6–13.
48. Keefe EB, Dieterich DT, Han SH, et al. A treatment algorithm for the management of chronic hepatitis B virus infection in the United States: 2008 update. Clin Gastroenterol Hepatol 2008;6:1315–41.
49. Thio CL. Hepatitis B and human immunodeficiency virus coinfection. Hepatology 2009;49:S138–45.
50. Kaplan JE, Benson C, Holmes KH, et al. Guidelines for prevention and treatment of opportunistic infections in HIV-infected adults and adolescents: recommendations from CDC, the National Institutes of Health, and the HIV Medicine Association of the Infectious Diseases Society of America. MMWR Morb Mortal Wkly Rep 2009;58:1.
51. Matthews GV, Dore GJ. Combination of tenofovir and lamivudine versus tenofovir after lamivudine failure for therapy of hepatitis B in HIV-coinfection. AIDS 2007;21: 777–8.
52. McMahon MA, Jilek BL, Brennan TP, et al. The HBV drug entecavir—effects on HIV-1 replication and resistance. N Engl J Med 2007;356:2614–21.
53. Chung RT, Andersen J, Volberding P, et al. Peginterferon alfa-2a plus ribavirin versus interferon alfa-2a plus ribavirin for chronic hepatitis C in HIV-coinfected persons. N Engl J Med 2004;351:451–9.
54. Delaugerre C, Marcelin AG, Thibault V, et al. Human immunodeficiency virus (HIV) type 1 reverse transcriptase resistance mutations in hepatitis B virus (HBV)-HIV-coinfected patients treated for HBV chronic infection once daily with 10 milligrams of adefovir dipivoxil combined with lamivudine. Antimicrob Agents Chemother 2002;46:1586.
55. Panel on Antiretroviral Guidelines for Adults and Adolescents. Guidelines for the use of antiretroviral agents in HIV-1-infected adults and adolescents. Bethesda (MD): Department of Health and Human Services; 2008. p. 1–139.
56. Hoofnagle JH. Reactivation of hepatitis B. Hepatology 2009;49:S156–65.
57. Yeo W, Chan PK, Zhong S, et al. Frequency of hepatitis B virus reactivation in cancer patients undergoing cytotoxic chemotherapy: a prospective study of 626 patients with identification of risk factors. J Med Virol 2000;62:299–307.
58. Lok AS, Liang RH, Chiu EK, et al. Reactivation of hepatitis B virus replication in patients receiving cytotoxic therapy. Report of a prospective study. Gastroenterology 1991;100:182–8.
59. Loomba R, Rowley A, Wesley R, et al. Systematic review: the effect of preventive lamivudine on hepatitis B reactivation during chemotherapy. Ann Intern Med 2008;148:519–28.
60. Yeo W, Zee B, Zhong S, et al. Comprehensive analysis of risk factors associating with Hepatitis B virus (HBV) reactivation in cancer patients undergoing cytotoxic chemotherapy. Br J Cancer 2004;90:1306–11.
61. Tur-Kaspa R, Shaul Y, Moore DD, et al. The glucocorticoid receptor recognizes a specific nucleotide sequence in hepatitis B virus DNA causing increased activity of the HBV enhancer. Virology 1988;167:630–3.

62. McMillan JS, Shaw T, Angus PW, et al. Effect of immunosuppressive and antiviral agents on hepatitis B virus replication in vitro. Hepatology 1995;22(1): 36–43.
63. Yeo W, Chan TC, Leung NW, et al. Hepatitis B virus reactivation in lymphoma patients with prior resolved hepatitis B undergoing anticancer therapy with or without rituximab. J Clin Oncol 2009;27(4):605–11.
64. Esteve M, Saro C, González-Huix F, et al. Chronic hepatitis B reactivation following infliximab therapy in Crohn's disease patients: need for primary prophylaxis. Gut 2004;53:1363–5.
65. Lau GK, Yiu HH, Fong DY, et al. Early is superior to deferred preemptive lamivudine therapy for hepatitis B patients undergoing chemotherapy. Gastroenterology 2003;125:1742–9.
66. Yeo W, Chan PK, Ho WM, et al. Lamivudine for the prevention of hepatitis B virus reactivation in hepatitis B s-antigen seropositive cancer patients undergoing cytotoxic chemotherapy. J Clin Oncol 2004;22:927–34.
67. Sumethkul V, Ingsathit A, Jirasiritham S. Ten-year follow-up of kidney transplantation from hepatitis B surface antigen-positive donors. Transplant Proc 2009;41(1): 213–5.
68. Lau GK, Leung YH, Fong DY, et al. High hepatitis B virus (HBV) DNA viral load as the most important risk factor for HBV reactivation in patients positive for HBV surface antigen undergoing autologous hematopoietic cell transplantation. Blood 2002;99:2324–30.
69. Fornairon S, Pol S, Legendre C, et al. The long-term virologic and pathologic impact of renal transplantation on chronic hepatitis B virus infection. Transplantation 1996;62(2):297–9.
70. Ridruejo E, Brunet Mdel R, Cusumano A, et al. HBsAg as predictor of outcome in renal transplant patients. Medicina (B Aires) 2004;64(5):429.
71. Harnett JD, Zeldis JB, Parfrey PS, et al. Hepatitis B disease in dialysis and transplant patients. Further epidemiologic and serologic studies. Transplantation 1987;44(3):369–76.
72. Lunel F, Cadranel JF, Rosenheim M, et al. Hepatitis virus infections in heart transplant recipients: epidemiology, natural history, characteristics, and impact on survival. Gastroenterology 2000;119(4):1064–74.
73. Wedemeyer H, Pethig K, Wagner D, et al. Long-term outcome of chronic hepatitis B in heart transplant recipients. Transplantation 1998;66(10):1347–53.
74. Magnone M, Holley JL, Shapiro R, et al. Interferon-alpha-induced acute renal allograft rejection. Transplantation 1995;59(7):1068–70.
75. Rakela J, Wooten RS, Batts KP, et al. Failure of interferon to prevent recurrent hepatitis B infection in hepatic allograft. Mayo Clin Proc 1989;64(4): 429–32.
76. Chan TM, Wu PC, Li FK, et al. Treatment of fibrosing cholestatic hepatitis with lamivudine. Gastroenterology 1998;115(1):177–81.
77. Liu CJ, Lai MY, Lee PH, et al. Lamivudine treatment for hepatitis B reactivation in HBsAg carriers after organ transplantation: a 4-year experience. J Gastroenterol Hepatol 2001;16(9):1001–8.
78. Rostaing L, Henry S, Cisterne JM, et al. Efficacy and safety of lamivudine on replication of recurrent hepatitis B after cadaveric renal transplantation. Transplantation 1997;64(11):1624–7.
79. Wang SS, Chou NK, Chi NH, et al. Successful treatment of hepatitis B virus infection with Lamivudine after heart transplantation. Transplant Proc 2006;38(7): 2138–40.

80. Potthoff A, Tillmann HL, Bara C, et al. Improved outcome of chronic hepatitis B after heart transplantation by long-term antiviral therapy. J Viral Hepat 2006; 13(11):734–41.

81. Gane E, Pilmore H. Management of chronic viral hepatitis before and after renal transplantation. Transplantation 2002;74(4):427–37.

82. Lau DT, Khokhar MF, Doo E, et al. Long-term therapy of chronic hepatitis B with lamivudine. Hepatology 2000;32(4 Pt 1):828–34.

83. Han DJ, Kim TH, Park SK, et al. Results on preemptive or prophylactic treatment of lamivudine in HBsAg (+) renal allograft recipients: comparison with salvage treatment after hepatic dysfunction with HBV recurrence. Transplantation 2001; 71(3):387–94.

84. Yeo W, Steinberg JL, Tam JS, et al. Lamivudine in the treatment of hepatitis B virus reactivation during cytotoxic chemotherapy. J Med Virol 1999;59(3):263–9.

85. Lau GK, Lie A, Liang R. Prophylactic lamivudine therapy for hepatitis B patients undergoing immunosuppressive therapy. Blood 2002;100(8):3054.

86. Chan TM, Fang GX, Tang CS, et al. Pre-emptive lamivudine therapy based on HBV DNA level in HBsAg-positive kidney allograft recipients. Hepatology 2002; 36(5):1246–52.

87. Liaw YF, Leung NW, Chang TT, et al. Effects of extended lamivudine therapy in Asian patients with chronic hepatitis B. Asia Hepatitis Lamivudine Study Group. Gastroenterology 2000;119(1):172–80.

88. Kohrt HE, Ouyang DL, Keeffe EB. Antiviral prophylaxis for chemotherapy-induced reactivation of chronic hepatitis B virus infection. Clin Liver Dis 2007; 11:965–91.

Hepatitis B Vaccination: Disease and Cancer Prevention—A Taiwanese Experience

Mei Hwei Chang, MD

KEYWORDS

- Hepatitis B virus • Hepatocellular carcinoma
- Hepatitis B vaccination • Hepatitis B immunoglobulin
- Hepatitis B surface antigen

Hepatitis B virus (HBV) infection is an important global health problem. It is a major cause of chronic hepatitis, liver cirrhosis, and hepatocellular carcinoma (HCC).[1] It is prevalent in Asia, Africa, southern Europe, and Latin America, where the hepatitis B surface antigen (HBsAg) seropositive rate ranges from 2% to 20%. Regions with a high prevalence of HBV infection also have high rates of HCC. HBV causes 60% to 80% of the primary liver cancer in the world, which accounts for 1 of the 3 major cancer deaths in Asia, the Pacific Rim, and Africa. In most parts of Asia, the HBsAg carrier rate in the general population is approximately 5% to 20%.[2,3] In highly prevalent areas such as Taiwan, primary HBV infections occur mainly during infancy and early childhood.[4] Before the implementation of the universal HBV vaccination program, the HBsAg seropositive (chronic HBV infection) rate in Taipei city increased with age, ranging from 5% in infants, to 10% in children at 2 years of age and remaining stationary afterward. This suggested that most chronic HBsAg carriers were infected before 2 years of age in endemic areas. In parts of Africa, such as rural Senegal, horizontal infection occurs very early. By the age of 2 years, 25% of children were infected, whereas at age 15, the infection rate was 80%.[5]

The age of primary infection is an important factor affecting the outcome. Infection during infancy and early childhood leads to high rates of chronicity.

Perinatal transmission from HBsAg carrier mothers to their infants is an important route of transmission leading to chronicity in endemic areas. Before the era of universal HBV vaccination, it accounts for the transmission route in 40% to 50% of

The author has nothing to disclose.
This work was supported by grants from the National Health Research Institute, Taiwan (Grant nos. NHRI-EX94-9418BI, NHRIEX95-9418BI, NHRI-EX96-9418BI, and NHRI-EX97-9418BI).
Department of Pediatrics, National Taiwan University Hospital, College of Medicine, National Taiwan University, No. 7, Chung-Shan S. Road, Taipei, Taiwan
E-mail address: changmh@ntu.edu.tw

HBsAg carriers in Asia. Status of maternal serum HBsAg and hepatitis B e antigen (HBeAg) affects the outcome of HBV infection in their infants. About 90% of the infants of HBeAg seropositive carrier mothers became HBsAg carriers (**Box 1**).[6] Horizontal transmission is from highly infectious family members, improperly sterilized syringes, or other contaminated instruments.[7,8] In Africa, HBV transmission was considered to occur mainly horizontally during early childhood.

UNIVERSAL HEPATITIS B VACCINATION PROGRAM

Immunoprophylaxis is the most cost-effective way to achieve global control of HBV infection and related complications.[9,10] The most important strategy has been the universal immunization program in infancy to prevent both perinatal and horizontal transmission of HBV infection. Passive immunization using hepatitis B immunoglobulin (HBIG) provides temporary immunity with high cost, whereas active immunization using vaccines provides long-term immunity and protection with lower expense.

Current programs for universal hepatitis B vaccination in infancy can be divided into 3 main strategies in the world depending on both the local epidemiologic conditions, ie, high or low prevalence rate of HBsAg carriage in children, and the budget of the government for HBV immunization.

Combined Passive and Active Immunization with Maternal Screening of HBsAg and HBeAg

In addition to active immunization with HBV vaccines, passive immunization with HBIG can neutralize HBV transmitted from the mother during the perinatal period. It must be given within 24 hours after birth. The world's first universal hepatitis B vaccination program was launched in July 1984 in Taiwan.[11] Pregnant women were screened for serum HBsAg and HBeAg. All infants received 4 doses (0, 1, 2, and 12 months of age) of plasma-derived HBV vaccine (before July 1992), or 3 doses (0, 1, and 6 months of age) of recombinant HBV vaccine (after July 1992). In addition, infants of high-risk mothers with positive HBeAg and HBsAg received 0.5 mL HBIG within 24 hours after birth. The expense of all the vaccines and HBIG given to the infants was covered by the government. The coverage rate of 3-dose hepatitis B vaccination for neonates was about 84% to 94%. The program was gradually extended to preschool and schoolchildren and adults.

Box 1
Effect of maternal serum HBV status on the outcome of HBV infection in their Infants

Maternal HBV status	Infant outcome	
	No vaccination	With immunoprophylaxis
HBeAg(+), HBsAg(−)	>90% chronicity	Vaccine + HBIG → 10%–15% chronic infection
HBeAg(−), HBsAg(+)	<5% chronicity, with risk of FH, AH	<1% chronic infection, with risk of FH, AH, but reduced
HBeAg(−), HBsAg(−)	Not infected	Not infected

Abbreviations: AH, acute hepatitis; FH, fulminant hepatitis; HBeAg, hepatitis B e antigen; HBsAg, hepatitis B surface antigen; HBIG, hepatitis B immunoglobulin.

Passive and Active Immunization with Maternal Screening of HBsAg

In countries like the United States, pregnant women were screened for HBsAg but not HBeAg. Every infant is recommended to receive 3 doses of HBV vaccines. In addition, all infants of HBsAg-positive mothers, regardless of the HBeAg status, received HBIG within 24 hours after birth.[12] This strategy saves the cost of maternal HBeAg screening, but increases the cost of HBIG, which is much more costly than the vaccine.

Active Immunization Without HBIG

In areas where HBV infection prevalence is low or financial resources are limited, immunization with 3 doses of HBV vaccine in a 0-, 1-, and 6-month schedule without antenatal screening of the mothers or administration of HBIG is a reasonable strategy to save cost. Such programs have been successful in Thailand and many other countries in Asia.[13]

THE EFFECT OF UNIVERSAL HEPATITIS B IMMUNIZATION ON THE CONTROL OF LIVER DISEASES AND HCC

HBV Vaccination Effectively Prevents HBV Infection

The incidence of chronic HBV infection in children has been reduced remarkably worldwide in areas where universal HBV vaccination has been introduced. Generally speaking, after the universal HBV vaccination program, the HBsAg seropositive rates were reduced to approximately one-tenth of the prevaccination rates. Serial epidemiologic surveys of HBV markers in Taipei city were conducted in 1984, 1989, 1994, 1999, and 2004 (before, and 5, 10, 15, and 20 years after the implementation of the vaccination program).[4,14–17] Twenty years after the launch of the universal HBV vaccination program, the HBsAg carrier rate decreased significantly from about 10% before the vaccination program to less than 1% afterward in vaccinated children younger than 20 years old. The total infection rate (acute and chronic infection) was also decreased, even in those who were not vaccinated during infancy. Anti-HBc seropositivity declined from 38.0% to 16.0% and further down to 4.6% in children 15 to 20 years after the program.[17]

In reports from many countries such as Gambia and Korea,[18,19] universal vaccination programs have been equally successful. The hepatitis B carrier rate has fallen from 5% to 10%, to less than 1%, demonstrating that universal vaccination is more effective than selective immunization for high-risk groups.

The Mortality Rate of Fulminant Hepatitis B is Reduced

HBV infection is the most important cause of fulminant hepatitis in children in areas hyperendemic for HBV infection. Infants are particularly susceptible to fulminant hepatitis B if the mother is seronegative for HBeAg but positive for HBsAg. The mortality rate is high (approximately 67%) in children with fulminant hepatitis B.[20] The mortality rate of fulminant hepatitis in infants born from 1974 to 1984 was 5.36 per 100,000 in Taiwan (before the HBV vaccination era). It was reduced to 1.71 per 100,000 from 1985 to 1998 (after the launch of HBV vaccination program), with a mortality ratio of 3.2 (P<.001).[21]

After the universal vaccination program in Taiwan, HBV was rarely the cause of fulminant hepatitis in children older than 1 year. Although the incidence of fulminant hepatitis B was reduced, it still remained as a major cause of fulminant hepatitis in infants. These infants were most likely perinatally infected from their HBeAg- negative HBsAg carrier mothers despite vaccination.[22]

Reduction of HCC After the Universal Vaccination Program

HCC in children is closely related to HBV infection and the characteristics are similar to HCC in adults.[23] In comparison with most other parts of the world, Taiwan has a high prevalence of HBV infection and HCC in children. Children with HCC in Taiwan are nearly 100% HBsAg seropositive, and most (86%) of them are HBeAg negative. Children with HCC are mostly (94%) maternal HBsAg positive.[23] The histologic findings of the tumor portion are similar to that in adult HCC. Most (80%) of the nontumor portion has liver cirrhosis. Integration of the HBV genome into the host genome was demonstrated in the HCC tissues in children.[24]

Current therapies for HCC are not satisfactory. Vaccination is the best way to prevent both precancerous and cancerous lesions of HCC; yet, the peak age of HCC in adults is about 40 to 60 years, and the effect of universal HBV vaccination in infancy on the reduction of adult HCC may require approximately 40 years to appear. The change of HCC incidence in children after the HBV vaccination era may reflect the future effect of HBV vaccination on HCC in adults.

The reduction in HBV infection after the launch of the universal hepatitis B vaccination program in July 1984 in Taiwan has had a dramatic effect on the reduction of HCC incidence in children. The annual incidence of HCC in children aged 6 to 14 was reduced from 0.52–0.54 per 100,000 children born before July 1984 to 0.13–0.20 per 100,000 children born after July 1984.[25–28]

The risk of developing HCC for vaccinated cohorts was statistically significantly associated with incomplete HBV vaccination, prenatal maternal HBsAg, or HBeAg seropositivity.[25–27] The prevention effect of HCC by HBV vaccine extends from childhood to early adulthood. Failure to prevent HCC results mostly from unsuccessful control of HBV infection by highly infectious mothers.[26–28]

Approximately 90% of the mothers of the children with HCC with known serum HBsAg status were positive for HBsAg. This provides strong evidence of perinatal transmission of maternal HBV as the main route of HBV transmission in children with HCC born after the immunization era, and was not effectively eliminated by the HBV immunization program.[27]

LONG-TERM IMMUNOGENICITY AND DURATION OF INFECTION PROTECTION

Long-term serial seroepidemiologic and immunologic studies of vaccinated children in Taiwan have provided evidence to support that universal HBV vaccination in infancy has provided adequate long-term protection for up to 20 years of age. HBV seromarkers were studied in 18,779 subjects from neonates to adults at 20 years following the world's first successful implementation of a universal HBV vaccination program for infants in Taiwan. The seropositive rates for HBsAg, anti-HBs, and anti-HBc were 1.2%, 50.5%, and 3.7%, respectively, in those younger than 20 years and born after the vaccination program.[4,14–17]

Although the vaccine remained highly efficacious in reducing the HBsAg positivity rate, 15 to 20 years after neonatal immunization with plasma-derived HBV vaccine, approximately 50% of children exhibited waning humoral immunity (anti-HBs <10 mIU/mL). It is estimated that 2% to 10% of the vaccinated population had lost their HBV vaccine-conferred booster response. This poses the potential risk of breakthrough infection.[29,30] However, the absence of an increase in HBsAg seropositive subjects at different ages in the same birth cohorts born after the vaccination program implies no actual increased risk of persistent HBV infection with age. A universal booster dose is not recommended for the primary HBV vaccinees in the general population before adulthood. (**Box 2**).[17]

A long-term follow-up study of 1200 vaccinated infants showed that no new HBsAg carrier occurs in vaccinees in spite of the loss of anti-HBs in part of the vaccinees. Anti-HBs was not detectable in 504 children at 7 years of age, and 200 of the 504 accepted a booster dose of HBV vaccine then. The annual anti-HBs disappearance rate was 10.2% during follow-up of 16-year-old children who did not receive a booster dose at age 7.[31,32]

A study of 493 Alaska Native persons who had received plasma-derived hepatitis B vaccine when older than 6 months also revealed that the protection in childhood or adulthood lasts at least 22 years. Booster doses are not needed. Considering persons with an anti-HBs level greater than or equal to 10 mIU/mL at 22 years and those who responded to 1 booster dose, protection was demonstrated in 87% of the participants. No new acute or chronic hepatitis B virus infections were identified.[33] Another study in Thailand followed 272 infants for 17 years after receiving 3 or 4 doses of HBV vaccine during infancy. Transient presence of HBsAg or transient and/or long-term presence of antibody to HBcAg suggested that this population was heavily exposed to HBV during the follow-up period, but no new cases of chronic HBV infection were observed. This study demonstrates the long-term protection effect of HBV vaccine in infancy without HBIG.[34]

Regarding the special high-risk group with HBV infection, such as recipients of liver transplantation, the titer of anti-HBs is recommended to be kept in a higher titer before transplantation. In the absence of adequate prophylaxis, the incidence of de novo HBV infection in pediatric orthotopic liver transplantation (OLT) recipients was reported to be 15% in a series of studies in Taiwan. An anti-HBs titer of greater than 200 mIU/mL before OLT may be sufficient to prevent de novo HBV infection in HBsAg-negative recipients.[35]

STRATEGIES TO REDUCE BREAKTHROUGH INFECTION AND NONRESPONDERS
Causes of Breakthrough Infection in Vaccines

Causes of breakthrough infection or nonresponders includes high maternal viral load,[36] intrauterine infection,[37,38] surface gene mutants, poor compliance, genetic hyporesponsiveness, and immunocompromised status (**Table 1**). A positive maternal HBsAg serostatus was found in 89% of the HBsAg seropositive subjects born after the launch of the HBV vaccination program in Taiwan. Maternal transmission is the primary reason for breakthrough HBV infection and is the challenge that needs to be addressed in future vaccination programs.[17] Appropriate HBIG administration for high-risk infants, efforts to minimize noncompliance, and new strategies to reduce breakthrough infections are needed.

Box 2
Recommendation for booster dose of HBV vaccine in vaccines

1. Universal booster is not recommended for children or adolescents with normal immune status.

2. For those with high risk of infection, if anti-HBs <10 mIU/mL, consider booster dose.

3. Boost immunocompromised persons when their anti-HBs <10 mIU/mL.

4. Keep anti-HBs >200 mIU/mL before receiving liver transplantation.

Table 1
Causes of breakthrough HBV infection in vaccinated children
1. Maternal factor High maternal viral titer Intrauterine infection
2. Viral factor Surface gene mutants
3. Host factor Genetic hyporesponsiveness Immune compromised host

During a long-term follow-up study from 7 to 16 years of age of vaccinated school children, HBsAg seropositive rates remained stationary at about 0.7% during the follow-up period from 7 to 16 years of age without development of new HBsAg carriers status during the follow-up period[31,32]; yet, new HBV infection, reflected by the annual anti-HBc seroconversion rate (with at least 2 anti-HBc positive samples 1 year apart), ranging from 0% to 0.4%, with a mean of 0.2%, did occur among vaccinees. None of the new anti-HBc seroconverters were seropositive for HBV DNA, nor became an HBsAg carrier. It suggests that horizontal transimissm is not a main cause leading to breakthrough chronic HBV infection in vaccinees.

Vaccine Escape Mutants—S Gene Mutants

The rate of HBsAg gene mutants in HBsAg carriers born after the vaccination program is increasing with time. The rate of HBV surface gene mutation was 7.8%, 17.8%, 28.1%, 23.8%, and 22.6% respectively among those seropositive for HBV DNA, at before, and 5, 10, 15, and 20 years after the launch of the HBV vaccination program.[39–41] The prevalence of HBV surface gene a determinant mutants in HBV DNA seropositive children with positive HBsAg or anti-HBc was higher in fully vaccinated than in unvaccinated children with seropositive HBV DNA. Fortunately, it remained stationary (22.6%) at 20 years after the vaccination program. HBV vaccine covering surface gene mutant proteins is still not urgently needed for routine HBV immunization at present, but careful and continuous monitoring for the surface gene mutants is needed.

Strategy Toward Successful Control of HBV Infection

Primary prevention by universal vaccination is most cost effective toward a successful control of HBV infection and its complications; yet currently there are several problems that remain to be solved (**Fig. 1**). The most important strategies of primary prevention for a better control of HBV infection globally include further increasing the world coverage rates of HBV vaccines, and better methods against breakthrough infection/nonresponsiveness. It is extremely important to find ways to reduce the cost of HBV vaccines, and to increase funding for HBV vaccination of children living in developing countries endemic of HBV infection. It is particularly urgent in areas where HBV infection and HCC are prevalent. Those who oppose HBV vaccination may be reduced in number by better communication and understanding of vaccine-related side effects. For instance, although there is little supporting evidence, an association between central nervous system demyelinating diseases and hepatitis B vaccine was suggested.[42] Clarification of the safety of the vaccines may help to reduce anxiety about the risks of the vaccine and enhance an appreciation of HBV vaccine benefits.

The World Health Organization (WHO) recommended that universal hepatitis B immunization should be introduced in all countries by the end of 1997. WHO also

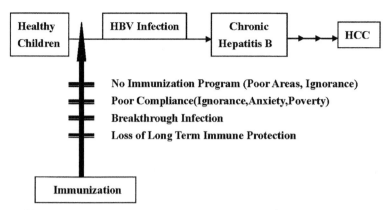

Fig. 1. Problems remain in vaccine prevention against HBV infection and related HCC.

established the objective to reduce the incidence of new HBV carriers among children by 80% by 2001.[43] Up to 2008, according to the report from WHO, approximately 71% (138 countries) of countries have followed this recommendation with a coverage rate of more than 80% for 3 doses of HBV vaccine. Efforts to further increase the coverage rates of HBV vaccines worldwide should be actively made. In spite of enormous achievement, progress of HBV immunization in most countries has been slow.[44] Increasing efforts are required to eliminate acute and chronic hepatitis B. Because of the competition of other new vaccines, HBV has not captured sufficient attention from policy makers, advocacy groups, or the general public. This is a major challenge for the future.[45] It is very important to persuade and support the policy makers of the countries that still have no universal HBV vaccination program to establish a program, and to encourage the countries that already have a program to increase the coverage rates. A comprehensive public health prevention program should include the prevention, detection, and control of HBV infections and related chronic liver diseases, and evaluation of the effectiveness of prevention activities.[46]

Further investigation into the mechanisms of breakthrough HBV infection or nonresponders is critical. Interventions to prevent perinatal or intrauterine infection, the development of HBV vaccines against surface antigen gene mutants, and better vaccines for immunocompromised individuals may further reduce the incidence of new HBV infections. Infants of HBsAg carrier mothers with positive HBeAg or high viral load are the high-risk group of breakthrough HBV infection, in spite of immunoprophylaxis with combination of passive (HBIG) and active (vaccine) immunization.

Nucleoside analog treatment during pregnancy was attempted to prevent perinatal transmission of HBV infection. Eight highly viremic (HBV DNA $\geq 1.2 \times 10^9$ copies/mL) mothers were treated with 150 mg of lamivudine per day during the last month (34 weeks) of pregnancy in a pilot study. All children received passive-active immunization at birth and were followed for 12 months. One (12.5%) of the 8 children in the lamivudine group and 7 (28%) of the 25 children in the historical control group were still HBsAg and HBV DNA positive at 12 months old.[47] Another clinical trial was conducted using entry criteria for mothers older than 16, with estimated gestational period of 26 to 30 weeks at screening, HBsAg positive, and serum HBV DNA above 1000 mEq/mL at screening.[48] Lamivudine 100 mg per day was given from 34 weeks of gestation to 4 weeks after delivery. Standard passive-active immunization was given to the infants. At week 52, 18% of the 56 infants of the lamivudine treatment group and 39% of the placebo group were HBsAg seropostive (*P* = .014). Unfortunately, 13% of the placebo group and 23% of the lamivudine group became lost to follow-up at week 52, which limited the interpretation of its primary analysis. Further studies to clarify the benefit and adverse reaction of nucleoside/nucleotide analogs in the prevention of intra-uterine/perinatal infection are needed.

CONCLUSIONS AND FUTURE PROSPECTS

Prevention is most cost effective toward successful control of HBV infection and its complications. It is particularly urgent in areas where HBV infection and HCC are prevalent. To achieve better results of primary HCC prevention globally, higher world coverage rates of HBV vaccine, better strategies against breakthrough infection/nonresponder, and good long-term protection are needed.

With the universal hepatitis B vaccination program starting from neonates in most countries, HBV infection and its complications will be further reduced in this century. It is expected that an effective decline in the incidence of HCC in adults will be achieved in the near future. The concept of a cancer preventive vaccine, using HBV as an example, can be applied further to other infectious agents and their related cancers.

REFERENCES

1. Ganem D, Prince AM. Hepatitis B virus infection natural history and clinical consequences. N Engl J Med 2004;350:1118–29.
2. Lavanchy D. Hepatitis B virus epidemiology, disease burden, treatment, and current and emerging prevention and control measures. J Viral Hepat 2004;11: 97–107.
3. Chang MH. Prospects for hepatitis B virus eradication and control of hepatocellular carcinoma. Baillieres Clin Gastroenterol 2000;13:511–7.
4. Hsu HY, Chang MH, Chen DS, et al. Baseline seroepidemiology of hepatitis B virus infection in children in Taipei, 1984: a study just before mass hepatitis B vaccination program in Taiwan. J Med Virol 1986;18:301–7.
5. Feret E, Larouze B, Dip B, et al. Epidemiology of hepatitis B virus infection in the rural community of Tip, Senegal. Am J Epidemiol 1987;125:140–9.
6. Stevens CE, Beasley RP, Tsui J, et al. Vertical transmission of hepatitis B antigen in Taiwan. N Engl J Med 1975;292:771–4.
7. Hsu SC, Chang MH, Ni YH, et al. Horizontal transmission of HBV in children. J Pediatr Gastroenterol Nutr 1993;16:66–9.
8. Beasley RP, Hwang LY, Lin CC, et al. Incidence of hepatitis B virus infection in preschool children in Taiwan. J Infect Dis 1982;146:198–204.
9. Beasley RP, Hwang LY, Stevens CE, et al. Efficacy of hepatitis B immune globulin for prevention of perinatal transmission of the hepatitis B virus carrier state: final report of a randomized double-blind, placebo-controlled trial. Hepatology 1983; 3:135–41.
10. Lee GC, Hwang LY, Beasley RP, et al. Immunogenicity of hepatitis B vaccine in healthy Chinese neonates. J Infect Dis 1983;148:526–9.
11. Chen DS, Hsu NH, Sung JL, et al. A mass vaccination program in Taiwan against hepatitis B virus infection in infants of hepatitis B surface antigen-carrier mothers. JAMA 1987;257:2597–603.
12. Shepard CW, Simard EP, Finelli L, et al. Hepatitis B virus infection: epidemiology and vaccination. Epidemiol Rev 2006;28:112–25.

13. Poovorawan Y, Theamboonlers A, Vimolket T, et al. Impact of hepatitis B immunization as part of the EPI. Vaccine 2000;19:943–9.
14. Tsen YJ, Chang MH, Hsu HY, et al. Seroepidemiology of hepatitis B virus infection in Taipei, 1989—Five years after a mass hepatitis B vaccination program. J Med Virol 1991;34:96–9.
15. Chen HL, Chang MH, Ni YH, et al. Seroepidemiology of hepatitis B virus infection in children—ten years of mass vaccination in Taiwan. J Am Med Assoc 1996;276: 906–8.
16. Ni YH, Chang MH, Huang LM, et al. Hepatitis B virus infection in children and adolescents in a hyperendemic area: 15 years after mass hepatitis B vaccination. Ann Intern Med 2001;135:796–800.
17. Ni YH, Huang LM, Chang MH, et al. Two decades of universal hepatitis B vaccination in Taiwan: impact and implication for future strategies. Gastroenterology 2007;132:1287–93.
18. Whittle HC, Maine N, Pilkington J, et al. Long-term efficacy of continuing hepatitis B vaccination in infancy in two Gambian villages. Lancet 1995;29(345):1089–92.
19. Jang MK, Lee JY, Lee JH, et al. Seroepidemiology of HBV infection in South Korea, 1995 through 1999. Korean J Intern Med 2001;16:153–9.
20. Chang MH, Lee CY, Chen DS, et al. Fulminant hepatitis in children in Taiwan: the important role of hepatitis B virus. J Pediatr 1987;111:34–9.
21. Kao JH, Hsu HM, Shau WY, et al. Universal hepatitis B vaccination and the decreased mortality from fulminant hepatitis in infants in Taiwan. J Pediatr 2001;139:349–52.
22. Chen HL, Chang CJ, Kong MS, et al. Fulminant hepatic failure in children in endemic area of hepatitis B virus infection: 15 years after universal hepatitis B vaccination. Hepatology 2004;39:58–63.
23. Chang MH, Chen DS, Hsu HC, et al. Maternal transmission of hepatitis B virus in childhood hepatocellular carcinoma. Cancer 1989;64:2377–80.
24. Chang MH, Chen PJ, Chen JY, et al. Hepatitis B virus integration in hepatitis B virus related hepatocellular carcinoma in childhood. Hepatology 1991;13:316–20.
25. Chang MH, Chen CJ, Lai MS, et al. Universal hepatitis B vaccination in Taiwan and the incidence of hepatocellular carcinoma in children. N Engl J Med 1997; 336:1855–9.
26. Chang MH, Shau WY, Chen CJ, et al. The effect of universal hepatitis B vaccination on hepatocellular carcinoma rates in boys and girls. JAMA 2000;284:3040–2.
27. Chang MH, Chen J, Hsu HM, et al. Prevention of hepatocellular carcinoma by universal vaccination against hepatitis B virus: the effect and problems. Clin Cancer Res 2005;11:7953–7.
28. Chang MH, You SL, Chen CJ, et al. Decreased incidence of hepatocellular carcinoma in hepatitis B vaccinees: a 20-year follow-up study. J Natl Cancer Inst 2009; 101:1348–55.
29. Lu CY, Ni YH, Chiang BL, et al. Humoral and cellular immune responses to a hepatitis B vaccine booster 15–18 years after neonatal immunization. J Infect Dis 2008; 197:1419–26.
30. Lu CY, Chiang BL, Chi WK, et al. Waning immunity to plasma-derived hepatitis B vaccine and the need for boosters 15 years after neonatal vaccination. Hepatology 2004;40:1415–20.
31. Lin YC, Chang MH, Ni YH, et al. Long-term immunogenicity and efficacy of universal hepatitis B virus vaccination in Taiwan. J Infect Dis 2003;187:134–8.
32. Wang CW, Wang LC, Chang MH, et al. Long-term follow-up of hepatitis B surface antibody levels in subjects receiving universal hepatitis B vaccination in infancy in

an area of hyperendemicity: correlation between radioimmunoassay and enzyme immunoassay. Clin Diagn Lab Imunol 2005;12:1442–7.

33. McMahon BJ, Dentinger CM, Bruden D, et al. Antibody levels and protection after hepatitis B vaccine: results of a 22-year follow-up study and response to a booster dose. J Infect Dis 2009;200:1390–6.

34. Poovorawan Y, Chongsrisawat V, Theamboonlers A, et al. Long-term benefit of hepatitis B vaccination among children in Thailand with transient hepatitis B virus infection who were born to hepatitis B surface antigen–positive mothers. J Infect Dis 2009;200:33–8.

35. Su WJ, Ho MC, Ni YH, et al. High-titer antibody to hepatitis B surface antigen before liver transplantation can prevent de novo hepatitis B infection. J Pediatr Gastroenterol Nutr 2009;48:203–8.

36. Lee SD, Lo KJ, Wu JC, et al. Prevention of maternal-infant hepatitis B virus transmission by immunization: the role of serum hepatitis B virus DNA. Hepatology 1986;6:369–73.

37. Tang JR, Hsu HY, Lin HH, et al. Hepatitis B surface antigenemia at birth: a long-term follow-up study. J Pediatr 1998;133:374–7.

38. Lin HH, Lee TY, Chen DS, et al. Transplacental leakage of HBeAg-positive maternal blood as the most likely route in causing intrauterine infection with hepatitis B virus. J Pediatr 1987;111:877–81.

39. Hsu HY, Chang MH, Liaw SH, et al. Changes of hepatitis B surface variants in carrier children before and after universal vaccination in Taiwan. Hepatology 1999;30:1312–7.

40. Hsu HY, Chang MH, Ni YH, et al. Survey of hepatitis B surface variant infection in children 15 years after nationwide vaccination program in Taiwan. Gut 2004;53: 1499–503.

41. Hsu HY, Chang MH, Ni YH, et al. Twenty-year trends in the emergence of hepatitis B surface antigen variants in children and adolescents after universal vaccination in Taiwan. J Infect Dis 2010;201:1192–200.

42. Halsey NA, Duclos P, van Damme P, et al. Hepatitis B vaccine and central nervous system demyelinating diseases. Viral Hepatitis Prevention Board. Pediatr Infect Dis J 1999;18:23–4.

43. WHO. Report on the Expanded Program on Immunization (EPI) of the World Health Organisation (WHO) Department of Vaccines and Biologicals. (Post-exposure immunization for hepatitis B). Available at: http://www.who.immunization. Accessed December 15, 2009.

44. Beasley RP. Rocks along the road to the control of HBV and HCC. Ann Epidemiol 2009;19:231–4.

45. Van Herck K, Vorsters A, Van Damme P. Prevention of viral hepatitis (B and C) reassessed. Best Pract Res Clin Gastroetenrol 2008;22:1009–29.

46. Lavanchy D. Chronic viral hepatitis as a public health issue in the world. Best Pract Res Clin Gastroenterol 2008;22:991–1008.

47. Van Zonneveld M, van Nunen AB, Niesters HGM, et al. Lamivudine treatment during pregnancy to prevent perinatal transmission of hepatitis B virus infection. J Viral Hepat 2003;10:294–7.

48. Xu WM, Cui YT, Wang L, et al. Efficacy and safety of lamivudine in late pregnancy for the prevention of mother-child transmission of hepatitis B: a multicentre, randomized, double-blind, placebo-controlled study. J Viral Hepat 2009;16: 94–103.

Chronic Hepatitis B: Past, Present, and Future

Michelle Lai, MD, MPH[a],*, Yun-Fan Liaw, MD[b]

KEYWORDS

• Hepatitis B virus • Vaccine • Screening

Before the discovery of the Australia antigen (Au-Ag) by Blumberg and coworkers,[1] progress in the understanding, prevention, and treatment of hepatitis B had been very slow. The link between hepatitis and Au-Ag in 1967[1] opened up a new era with unprecedented advances in the understanding and control of hepatitis B virus (HBV) infection. The goal of full implementation of national vaccination programs is still not within reach. Although currently there is effective therapy to suppress viral replication, there remains a great deal to be accomplished in the areas of prevention, screening, and treatment. This article discusses the past, present, and future perspective of HBV infection. The past perspective covers the first three decades following the discovery of Au-Ag; the present perspective spans the period from the approval of the first oral antiviral agent (1998) to the present. The future perspective discusses future challenges and directions.

PAST PERSPECTIVE: FIRST THREE DECADES AFTER THE DISCOVERY
Development of Diagnostic Tests for HBV

Five years after the discovery of Au-Ag, Dane and coworkers[2] discovered the complete hepatitis virion (Dane particle) by electron microscopy. In 1971, Almeida and coworkers[3] applied detergent to Dane particle and found an outer coat of Au-Ag and an inner component or core particle under immune electron microscopy. The particles were later known to be hepatitis B surface antigen (HBsAg) and core antigen (HBcAg), respectively. Au-Ag was renamed as HBsAg. By 1975, it was found that the core of the virion contains DNA and DNA polymerase.[4,5] By 1980, the genome of the virus had been sequenced.[6] Since early 1980s, the development of assays for

[a] Department of Medicine, Division of Gastroenterology, Beth Israel Deaconess Medical Center, Harvard University, 110 Francis Street, Suite 8E, Boston, MA 02215, USA
[b] Liver Research Unit, Chang Gung Memorial Hospital, Chang Gung University College of Medicine, 199, Tung Hwa North Road, Taipei 105, Taiwan
* Corresponding author.
E-mail address: mlai@bidmc.harvard.edu

Clin Liver Dis 14 (2010) 531–546
doi:10.1016/j.cld.2010.05.003
1089-3261/10/$ – see front matter © 2010 Elsevier Inc. All rights reserved.

HBV DNA and DNA polymerase has allowed the analysis of virus level in the blood and liver tissue.[7-9]

The discovery of viral particles allowed for worldwide seroprevalence study and the screening of blood supplies. Screening of donated blood for HBsAg was introduced in 1971. Screening for antibody to HBcAg (anti-HBc) began in 1987 as a surrogate assay for carriers of non-A, non-B hepatitis. The test was shown to detect some HBsAg-negative donors who are capable of transmitting HBV. In 1990, the anti-HBc assay was licensed by the Food and Drug Administration (FDA) based on its ability to decrease the risk of HBV infection. IgM anti-HBc allowed for the diagnosis of acute HBV infection.

A third antigen, the e antigen (HBeAg), and antibody to this antigen (anti-HBe), were first described in 1972 by Magnius and Espmark.[10] HBeAg is associated primarily with the core antigen in the virus's internal structure and is secreted from the hepatocytes and circulates in serum.[11] Multiple studies over subsequent years established the seropositivity for HBeAg as a marker of active viral replication, infectivity of the patient's serum, and predictor of chronic liver disease.[11-22] The availability of the assay for HBeAg and anti-HBe allowed for better understanding of the natural history of chronic HBV infection, including the different phases of immune tolerance, immune clearance, and residual or inactive state. The character-ization of hepatitis A, C, and D viruses over the next decades led to the develop-ment of assays for antibodies against these viruses. The availability of these assays allowed for diagnosis of concurrent infections in hepatitis B patients.

Development of Hepatitis B Vaccines

Soon after the discovery of Au-Ag, an effective HBV vaccine was developed. Almost simultaneously, both the Merck Institute of Medical Research in the United States and the Institute Pasteur in Paris independently developed a plasma-derived vaccine composed of HBsAg, which eventual became commercially available. Clinical trials of these vaccines were conducted first in European adults and African children in the mid-1970s,[23,24] and then male homosexuals in New York in the late 1970s.[25] In 1981, the FDA approved the first commercially available HBV vaccine. In the mid-1980s, recombinant HBV vaccines were introduced, eliminating the potential to trans-mit blood-borne infections. A combination vaccine (Twinrix, GlaxoSmithKline), including Energix-B and HAVRIX (hepatitis A vaccine) was approved by the FDA in May 2001.[26]

In the late 1970s, the hepatitis B immunoglobulin (HBIg) became available, resulting in drastically improved outcomes for chronic hepatitis B patients posttransplantation, decreasing the risk of perinatal transmission, and decreasing transmission rates with needlesticks when used as postexposure prophylaxis.[27]

Following the HBV vaccine trials in Taiwan, a country where HBV is highly endemic, the world's first HBV universal vaccination program was launched on July 1, 1984. In the first 2 years of the program, newborns of HBsAg-carrier mothers were vaccinated. Vaccination was extended to all newborns in July 1986 and to preschool children in July 1987. In 1988, the vaccination program was expanded to cover school children, teenagers, and then adults. In addition to the HBV vaccine, newborns of HBsAg-carrier mothers were also given HBIg within 24 hours after birth.[28]

Universal vaccination of all newborns was recommended in the United States in 1991. Integration of the HBV vaccine into national immunization programs was recom-mended by the Global Advisory Group of the Expanded Program on Immunization the same year and endorsed by the World Health Organization in May 1992. This recom-mendation set 1995 as a target date for countries with a HBV carrier prevalence of 8%

or higher, and 1997 as the target date for all other countries. In 1994, the World Health Assembly added a disease reduction target for hepatitis B, calling for an 80% decrease in new HBV carrier children by 2001.

Understanding Natural History

The development of HBV assays has allowed worldwide study on the prevalence and sequelae of HBV infection. Studies in Taiwan in 1970s demonstrated that HBV infection acquired perinatally or during early infancy or childhood contributed to 40% to 50% of chronic HBV infection in hyperendemic area, and the rate of chronicity reduced with increasing age at the time of HBV infection.[29]

The natural course of chronic hepatitis B infection was divided into replicative, HBeAg-positive and nonreplicative, HBeAg-negative phases before the mid-1980s.[30] After Chu and colleagues[30,31] published their clinicopathologic study using both HBeAg and HBV DNA assays, chronic HBV infection was reconceptualized as three phases: (1) immune-tolerant phase, (2) immune-clearance phase, and (3) residual or inactive phase. It was suggested that younger patients who were HBeAg seropositive with high viral loads ($>2 \times 10^{6-7}$ IU/mL or $>10^7$–10^8 copies/mL), normal serum aminotransferase (ALT), and near normal liver histology were in the immune-tolerant phase.[30,32] A long immune-tolerant phase is typically seen in Asian patients with chronic HBV infection acquired perinatally or in early childhood, whereas this phase is not apparent or very short in patients who acquired HBV infection during childhood.[32] Immune-clearance phase, in contrast, is characterized by intermittent or continuing hepatitis activity or episodic acute flares (serum ALT over five times the upper limit of normal [ULN]) that can be complicated by risk of hepatic decompensation. The immune-clearance phase can result in either disease progression or lead to HBeAg seroconversion to anti-HBe or undetectable HBV DNA, which occurs at an annual rate of 2% to 15%, depending on age, gender, baseline ALT, and severity of hepatitis.[33] After spontaneous HBeAg seroconversion, patients enter a remission or inactive phase with low serum HBV DNA (<2000 IU/mL) and normal ALT.[34,35] Following a long period of sustained remission after HBeAg seroconversion, spontaneous HBsAg seroclearance may occur at an annual rate of 0.5% to 2%, depending on age, HBV genotype, and underlying disease state.[36–39] In the early 1980s, HBeAg-negative HBV DNA–positive chronic active hepatitis was described as a major form of chronic hepatitis B in Europe.[40–42] It was shown to be caused by HBV with precore or basal core promoter mutations that abolish or down-regulate the translation of HBeAg.[41]

Studies showed that both patients with HBeAg-positive or HBeAg-negative hepatitis had an 2% to 4% annual incidence of cirrhosis.[34,35,43] Risk factors for progression to cirrhosis include male gender, frequency and severity of hepatitis, or liver injuries.[34,35,43] Once cirrhosis develops, patients are at risk for further disease progression to hepatic decompensation, hepatocellular carcinoma (HCC), or death.[36] The incidence of HCC was estimated to be less than 1% per year in cohorts of patients with chronic hepatitis B,[44] and increased to 3% to 6% in cohorts of patients with various stage of liver cirrhosis.[45]

HBV Replication, Pathogenesis, and Treatment

Besides advances in detection and prevention over this time period, the life cycle of HBV replication and pathogenesis of liver injuries were also elucidated. It was recognized that covalently closed circular DNA (cccDNA) is the template of hepatitis B virus transcription, and nuclear cccDNA accumulated in hepatocyte nuclei played a key role in the maintenance of chronic HBV infection.[46] Liver injury and ALT elevations were shown to be the result of the host's immune response against HBV, such as HLA class I antigen restricted, cytotoxic T-lymphocyte mediated hepatocytolysis.[47]

The first treatment for chronic hepatitis B, interferon alfa-2b (IFN-α), was evaluated in 1980s and was approved by the FDA for hepatitis in 1991. It was shown that conventional IFN-α therapy resulted in sustained response only in 30% to 40% of HBeAg-positive patients and 15% to 20% in HBeAg-negative patients.[48] Long-term benefit of IFN therapy was also demonstrated in terms of reduction in fibrosis progression, decrease in cirrhosis and HCC development, and prolonged survival, especially in sustained responders.[49]

PRESENT PERSPECTIVES: RECENT 10 YEARS
Impact of Mass HBV Vaccination

As of December 2007, 171 countries have introduced hepatitis B vaccine into their national immunization program. The estimated global third dose HBV vaccine coverage for infants, however, was only 60% in 2006.[50] The efficacy of mass immunization in decreasing HBV carrier rate is clearly shown by the Taiwanese experience. After 20 years into the vaccination program in Taiwan, the HBV carrier rate among children younger than 15 years of age has decreased from 9.8% at the start of the program to 0.5% in 2004.[51] Anti-HBc prevalence in the age cohort born before the vaccination program was 20.6% compared with 2.9% among the age cohort born after the implementation of the vaccination program. Along with the decrease in HBV infection, average annual hepatitis mortality rate in infants before and after the vaccination program decreased from 5.36 to 1.71 per 100,000 in the population.[52] Chen and colleagues[53] found that after vaccination, HBV-positive fulminant hepatic failure was rare in children greater than 1 year old, but was prone to develop in infants born to HBeAg-negative, HBsAg-carrier mothers. The infants who developed HBV-positive fulminant hepatic failure had not received HBIg according to the vaccination program in place. These findings clearly demonstrate that universal vaccination can control vertical and horizontal transmission of HBV infection. As seen in Taiwan, other countries that have adopted this recommendation have experienced a marked reduction in carrier rates. This has been most evident in regions with a high prevalence of chronic HBV. The reduction in carrier rates ranged from 16% before implementation of the program to 0% after implementation in Alaska, 7% to 0.5% in Samoa, and 12% to 3% in Micronesia.[54]

This decreased carrier rate with an aggressive vaccination program has resulted in decreased incidence of HCC.[51,53,55,56] In a landmark study, Chang and colleagues[55] from Taiwan showed that universal vaccination against hepatitis B was associated with a more than 50% decline in the incidence of HCC among children. The incidence of childhood HCC has decreased from 1.02 and 0.48 per 100,000 male and female children, respectively, to 0.3 and 0.18 per 100,000 male and female children, respectively. The most recent data have shown a decrease in the incidence of HCC in young adults of age 15 to 19 from 0.6 to 0.16 per 100,000.[56]

Impact of Assays for HBV DNA and Genotypes

Other important developments that arose out of HBV polymerase chain reaction (PCR) techniques were the improvement of HBV DNA assay and HBV genotyping. Since 1999, more and more sensitive commercial HBV DNA assays with varying limits of detection and dynamic range were developed successively. PCR-based assays have improved sensitivity and wider range of detection. Real-time PCR-based assays (eg, COBAS Taqman, RealART HBV, and Abbott Real Time PCR) are both sensitive and reliable over a broad range of detection. COBAS Taqman HBV test was the first hepatitis B viral load quantification assay to be approved by the FDA, in September of 2008. The development of ultrasensitive HBV DNA tests allowed for the study of HBV DNA levels as predictors of long-term outcomes, such as progression to cirrhosis and development of HCC.[57,58] The ability to quantify HBV DNA also allowed for monitoring response to treatment, once the treatments were available.

The development of assays for HBV genotypes (A–H) has led to further understanding of the epidemiology, biology, and pathology of HBV and the natural history of chronic HBV infection.[59] Compared with genotype B, it has been shown that genotype C HBV infection is associated with delayed HBeAg seroconversion, more frequent HBV reactivation, and higher risk of disease progress to cirrhosis or HCC. Genotyping is used to individualize therapy by predicting response to specific therapies and likelihood of HCC and detecting resistance mutations.

These assays have allowed for better understanding of the natural history of chronic HBV infection. Some of the patients who remain HBsAg seropositive with remission after HBeAg seroconversion can relapse back to active hepatitis at an annual incidence of 1.5% to 3.3%,[34,35,37] with higher rates in male, genotypes C or D infected patients, and those who HBeAg seroconverted after age 40.[35,60,61] The risk of relapse is significantly lower in young patients (age <30) with an annual incidence of 0.9%.[37] The relapse back to active hepatitis is caused by reactivation of either wild-type HBV (HBeAg seroreversion) or HBV with precore or basal core promoter mutations that abolish or down-regulate the production of HBeAg.[34,35] Such patients have a high risk of progression to cirrhosis and HCC.[57] In contrast, the risk is extremely low in patients with normal serum ALT in the immune-tolerant phase or inactive phase.[62,63] Recent large cohort long-term follow-up studies have shown that HBsAg seroclearance is usually associated with excellent prognosis.[64] HCC still occurs at a very low rate, however, and usually in those individuals who had already developed cirrhosis or superinfection with other viruses before the HBsAg clearance.

Current Anti-HBV Therapy

The approval of lamivudine, the first oral antiviral therapy for HBV, in 1998 has revolutionized the therapy of chronic HBV. In addition, the last several years has seen the FDA approval of an additional five therapies (**Table 1**). Currently approved therapies for chronic HBV infection include standard IFN, pegylated (Peg) IFN-α2a, and five nucleoside or nucleotide analogs: (1) lamivudine, (2) adefovir, (3) entecavir, (4) telbivudine, and (5) tenofovir. Oral antiviral agents have fast and potent inhibitory effects on HBV polymerase and reverse transcriptase activity, and are safe and effective for HBV

Table 1
FDA-approved treatment for chronic hepatitis B infection

Drug Name	Mechanism	FDA Approval
Intron A (interferon alfa-2b)	Immunomodulator	1991
Epivir-HBV (lamivudine)	Inhibits viral DNA polymerase	1998
Hepsera (adefovir dipivoxil)	Inhibits viral DNA polymerase	2002
Pegasys (peginterferon alfa-2a)	Immunomodulator	2005
Baraclude (entecavir)	Inhibits viral DNA polymerase	2005
Tyzeka (telbivudine; Sebivo, Europe)	Inhibits viral DNA polymerase	2006
Viread (tenofovir)	Inhibits viral DNA polymerase	2008

DNA suppression, ALT normalization, and histologic improvement. Most importantly, oral antiviral therapy has led to increased survival of acute fulminant hepatitis B,[65] drastic improvement in outcomes of patients suffering from hepatic decompensation, decreased rates of hepatic decompensation, and decreased need for liver transplantation.[66] This is particularly important in patients about to receive chemotherapy or immunosuppression agent.[67] The antiviral potency of these drugs does not result in an increase in HBeAg seroconversion, however, which was seen at a rate of around 20% after 1 year of treatment, and HBsAg loss is very rare. Continuing long-term drug therapy is usually necessary to maintain a virologic response. The emergence of drug-resistant genotypic mutations of HBV in long-term therapy is a major problem. Rescue therapy for drug resistance is now available.

Besides decreasing the need for liver transplantation, lamivudine was shown to improve outcomes further for patients with chronic hepatitis B posttransplantation when added to HBIg. Samuel and colleagues[68] in 1993 demonstrated that the use of HBIg as posttransplantation prophylaxis decreased the hepatitis B recurrence rate from 75% to 36%. Fischer and colleagues[69] showed that the addition of lamivudine to HBIg further decreased posttransplantation recurrent hepatitis B to 0.9%. Graft survival increased from 25% with HBIg alone to 92% with lamivudine and HBIg. There are also data to suggest that a lower dose of HBIg is needed with the addition of oral antiviral agent.[70]

Maintenance antiviral therapy has also led to improvement in long-term outcomes of chronic hepatitis B, such as the ability to reduce fibrosis progression, reverse fibrosis, reduce hepatic decompensation, and reduce the risk of HCC.[71–74] A randomized double-blind placebo-controlled trial showed significant difference in outcomes between the two groups.[74] An increase in Child-Pugh score greater than or equal to two was seen in 3.4% of the lamivudine group versus 8.8% in the placebo group. HCC occurred in 3.9% in the lamivudine group versus 7.4% in the placebo group.

Peg IFN was shown to be better than conventional IFN in terms of HBeAg response and once weekly administration.[75] Phase III trials have shown sustained response to 1-year Peg IFN-α2a, 180 mg once weekly, in 32% of HBeAg-positive patients and 43% of HBeAg-negative patients, with 3% HBsAg loss, and that combination with lamivudine had no added efficacy.[76,77]

Despite these advances, the currently available HBV therapies are far from satisfactory. Problems with current drug therapy include low therapy-induced HBeAg seroconversion rate, unpleasant side effect profile of IFN-based therapy, HBV virologic relapse after short-term nucleotide analogue therapy, drug resistance on prolonged nucleotide analogue therapy, and inability to completely eradicate HBV. The high cost of medical care and antiviral treatment is also a barrier to both diagnosis and treatment of diagnosed patients in some parts of the world.[78,79] Because of these problems, the treatment of chronic HBV requires individualized assessment and decision. This includes on-treatment response prediction and adjustment according to levels of HBsAg, HBeAg, or HBV DNA.[79]

Consensus

To address the complexity of management for patients with chronic HBV, several treatment guidelines have been put forth by panels of experts, including guidelines by American Association for the study of liver diseases (AASLD), European Association for the Study of the Liver (EASL), Asian Pacific Association for the study of the liver (APASL), and Keefe and colleagues.[80–83] Although these guidelines concur on certain management strategies, they disagree on others.

These guidelines agree on the screening for chronic hepatitis B and vaccination of all high-risk patients (**Table 2**). They also agree that the following chronic hepatitis B patients should be treated: (1) decompensated cirrhosis, (2) compensated cirrhosis and HBV DNA greater than 2000 IU/mL, and (3) noncirrhotic patients with significant level of HBV DNA (>20,000 IU/mL for HBeAg-positive patients and >2000 IU/mL in HBeAg-negative patients) and ALT greater than two times ULN. Peg IFN, entecavir, and tenofovir are recommended as first-line therapy in noncirrhotic patients, and entecavir or tenofovir in cirrhotic patients. At this time, experts agree that there are not enough data to support the use of de novo combination antiviral therapy.[80,81,83] Recent data have demonstrated that the true normal values of ALT are significantly lower than previously established limits of 40 to 65 IU/mL.[84,85] Some guidelines propose lowering the ULN value,[80,83] whereas others propose distinguishing between low normal ALT ($\leq$0.5 times ULN) and high normal ALT (0.5–1 times ULN).[82] There is still much controversy and debate over the management of chronic hepatitis B in certain groups of patients. Practices vary from provider to provider, and recommendations vary from guideline to guideline.

Controversies and Debates

There is disagreement on the management of noncirrhotic patients with normal ALT or mildly elevated ALT (one to two times ULN). The APASL and AASLD guidelines

Table 2
Screening recommendations for chronic hepatitis B and hepatocellular carcinoma

Screening for	Chronic Hepatitis B	HCC in Patients with Chronic Hepatitis B
Recommended in	Persons born in high or intermediate endemic areas	Asian men >40 years old
	United States–born persons not vaccinated as infants whose parents were born in regions with high HBV endemicity	Asian women >50 years old
	Persons with chronically elevated aminotransferases	Persons with cirrhosis
	Persons needing immunosuppressive therapy	Persons with a family history of HCC
	Men who have sex with men	Africans >20 years old
	Persons with multiple sexual partners or history of sexually transmitted disease	Any carrier >40 years old with persistent or intermittent ALT elevation or high HBV DNA level >2000 IU/mL
	Inmates of correctional facilities Persons who have ever used injecting drugs Dialysis patients HIV- or HCV-infected individuals Pregnant women Family members, household members, and sexual contacts of HBV-infected persons	
Screening method	Serum hepatitis B surface antigen and anti-HBs	Serum alphafetoprotein and ultrasound every 3–6 months or 6–12 months

Abbreviation: HCV, hepatitis C virus.

recommend close monitoring in noncirrhotic patients with normal or mildly elevated ALT levels, whereas the EASL and Keeffe and colleagues[80] guidelines have a lower threshold for liver biopsy and treatment (**Table 3**). APASL and Keefe and colleagues[80] recommend consideration of liver biopsy in older patients (age >35–40 years) with significant viral load and normal or high normal ALT, respectively, whereas EASL and AASLD recommend liver biopsy in patients with elevated ALT or ALT one to two times ULN, respectively. The recommendations by APASL and Keeffe and colleagues[80] are based on recent data that up to one third of patients with chronic hepatitis B and persistently normal ALT can have significant inflammation or fibrosis.[86–89] The risk factors for significant fibrosis are increasing age (>35–40 years); higher ALT level (26–40 IU/mL); and HBeAg positivity.

The APASL guidelines provide evidence to recommend IFN-based therapy in patients with well-compensated cirrhosis who may have an even better response than their non-cirrhotic counterparts.[45] They also suggest that oral antiviral therapy can be stopped if HBV DNA has been undetected for greater than 12 months during therapy.[82]

FUTURE PERSPECTIVE

Over the last few decades, advances in the field of hepatitis B have resulted in understanding of the natural history of chronic HBV infection, effective vaccines against the virus, sensitive assays for screening and monitoring of treatment, and effective treatments for viral suppression, all leading to improved outcomes. There is still much work, however, to be done. We are still far from the goal of full implementation of national vaccination programs. Although currently there are effective therapies to suppress viral replication, there remains a great deal to be accomplished in the coming years in the areas of prevention, screening, and treatment. As discussed, the vaccination rate in most endemic countries is abysmally low. Notably, worldwide, there are still 400 million people living with chronic hepatitis B and approximately 600,000 die annually from complications of hepatitis B.

PREVENTION

Despite overwhelming evidence of the benefits of universal vaccination, adoption of the national immunization program has not always translated to successful implementation of the program. Data collected from the World Health Organization and the United Nations Children's Fund showed that only 27% of newborns worldwide received a hepatitis B vaccine birth dose in 2006. In the 87 countries with greater than or equal to 8% chronic HBV infection prevalence, hepatitis B vaccine birth dose coverage was only 36%.[90] The need to implement this key hepatitis B prevention strategy more widely is apparent.

Hepatitis B vaccination programs need to be assigned higher priority and given more resources to prevent new infections. Financial resources need to be allocated for vaccination in lower-income countries. In addition, setting up clean needle exchange programs will also decrease the number of new infections. An intranasal HBV vaccine consisting of the surface and core antigen of HBV has been developed and is undergoing study to determine safety and efficacy. Although an intranasal vaccine may potentially increase vaccine use in countries where parenteral administration is not readily available, the cost of the vaccine will be a factor in its use.

Awareness and Active Screening

Most patients with chronic HBV infection have few or no symptom, and thus largely remain undiagnosed. A survey of 3163 Asian-American adults showed that only

Table 3
Guideline recommendations on management of patient with chronic HBV

	AASLD	APASL	EASL	Keefe et al[80]
Liver biopsy	HBeAg+, ALT persistently 1–2 × ULN or age >40 HbeAg−, HBV DNA 2000–20,000 IU/mL, ALT persistently 1–2 × ULN	Detectable HBV DNA and ↑ALT High normal ALT and age >40	↑ALT or HBV DNA >2000 IU/mL	Normal ALT if age >35–40 and HBV DNA ≥20,000 IU/mL in HBeAg+ ≥2000 IU/mL in HBeAg−
Treatment				
HBeAg+ patients	ALT persistently >2 × ULN Moderate or greater inflammation or fibrosis on biopsy	HBV DNA ≥20,000 IU/mL and ALT >2 × ULN If persistently elevated or concern about hepatic decompensation or Moderate or greater inflammation or fibrosis on biopsy	HBV DNA >2000 IU/mL or ALT >1 × ULN and Moderate or greater inflammation or fibrosis on biopsy	HBV ≥20,000 IU/mL ALT >1 × ULN
HBeAg− patients	ALT ≥2 × ULN and HBV DNA ≥20,000 IU/mL Moderate or greater inflammation or fibrosis on biopsy	HBV-DNA ≥2000 IU/mL and ALT persistently >2 × ULN, or concerns of hepatic decompensation Moderate or greater inflammation or fibrosis on biopsy		HBV ≥2000 IU/mL ALT >1 × ULN
Patients with cirrhosis	Decompensated Compensated *HBV DNA >2000 IU/mL *HBV DNA <2000 IU/mL if ↑ALT	Decompensated	Decompensated Compensated and HBV DNA >2000 IU/mL	Decompensated Compensated and detectable HBV DNA

35% of the chronically infected persons were aware that they were infected.[91] Another survey in Korean-Americans showed cirrhosis in 11% of the incidentally detected HBsAg-positive persons.[92] The situation in less-developed countries may be worse.[79] Detection of these asymptomatic HBsAg carriers requires active screening programs, especially in high-risk populations. In this regard, awareness among health care practitioners and governments is very important. This requires educating primary care physicians, internists, gastroenterologists, and even hepatologists. In many countries, lack of specialist and state-of art laboratory assays is also a serious problem. Future developments in noninvasive methods (serum and biophysical) of evaluation will allow easier and more widespread assessment of patients with chronic HBV to determine the severity of liver disease and monitor progression.

Even in the highly developed United States, a committee of the Institute of Medicine[93] recently confirmed the previous findings. They concluded that there is a lack of knowledge and awareness about chronic viral hepatitis on the part of health care and social-service providers, and among at-risk populations, members of the public, and policy-makers. Because of the insufficient understanding about the extent and seriousness of this public-health problem, inadequate public resources are being allocated to prevention, control, and surveillance programs. They make multiple important recommendations to improve surveillance, knowledge and awareness, and vaccination of HBV. The recent introduction of the Viral Hepatitis and Liver Cancer Control and Prevention Act 2009 (H.R. 3974) in the US congress is an important step.

Future Treatment Strategies

After patients at risk for developing complications from HBV are identified, improving treatment strategies to achieve better viral suppression and ultimately viral eradication and effective HCC surveillance are vital to reducing morbidity and mortality. There are now newer and more potent antiviral agents with high genetic barrier to drug resistance. Drugs with low genetic barrier are still widely used, however, in low-income countries where cost and reimbursement are critical issues.[79] An important goal of future treatment strategies is to overcome drug resistance in such a situation. By shortening the duration of treatment by achieving early response end point, the risk of drug resistance can be decreased. To achieve this end, physicians need to be educated on when and in whom appropriate therapy should be initiated.[82,94] Application of a road-map concept of approach may also reduce the cost.[78,95–97] For Peg IFN, a randomized control trial is ongoing to determine whether a lower dose or a shorter duration or both are still optimal for the therapy of chronic hepatitis B.

In addition to education of community clinicians, there is a great deal to be done to improve treatment strategies. Knowledge of natural history, especially in immunotolerant patients, needs to be improved, and the role of HBV genotype in determining prognosis elucidated. New therapeutic approaches, including new agents, combination therapy, and immunomodulatory therapies, should be assessed and aimed at decreasing drug resistance rate, increasing HBeAg and HBsAg seroconversion rate, and eradicating cccDNA. There is also the need to assess long-term impact of therapy on the prevention of cirrhosis and its complications, including HCC.

Currently available Nucleoside Analogues (NAs) are aimed at inhibition of viral replication but are not able to achieve viral eradication. Potential future targets of therapy are blocking HBV cell entry, HBV open reading frame transcription, viral packaging, HBV secretion, and cccDNA clearance. The presence of cccDNA in patients with occult hepatitis B (negative HBsAg) accounts for reactivation of hepatitis B in the setting of immunosuppression. Werle-Lapostolle and colleagues[98] showed that cccDNA loads vary significantly in different phases of chronic hepatitis B infection and that patients who underwent HBeAg seroconversion were more likely to have lower cccDNA levels at the beginning of therapy. Currently, there is limited understanding of the factors regulating the transcriptional activity of cccDNA. More work is needed in this area to achieve cure of hepatitis B instead of control of HBV replication.

Other potential future therapies include adoptive transfer of immunity and gene therapy. Adoptive transfer of immunity is the transfer of cells with immune memory against a given pathogen (ie, HBV). This could be used in liver transplant recipients in whom bone marrow or peripheral lymphocytes transferred from immunized donors can cause seroconversion to anti-HBs. These cells may even eradicate pre-existing HBV from transplant recipients.[99] A related strategy is the transfer of cytotoxic T cells primed in vitro with specific HBV peptide antigens. These transferred cytotoxic T cells would then eliminate hepatocytes that developed HBV infection posttransplantation.[99] Because of the immune attack on HBV-infected cells, this therapy does have the potential danger of causing severe hepatocellular necrosis.[99] Potential gene therapy would involve targeted delivery of specifically constructed DNA and RNA sequences that can integrate into HBV nuclear processes and disrupt viral replication.[100]

SUMMARY

There have been tremendous advances in the field of HBV-related disease. Great progress has been made in the understanding, prevention, and management of HBV. There is still a great deal to be accomplished, however, and there seems a long way to go before eradication of HBV infection.

REFERENCES

1. Blumberg BS, Gerstley BJ, Hungerford DA, et al. A serum antigen (Australia antigen) in Down's syndrome, leukemia, and hepatitis. Ann Intern Med 1967; 66:924–31.
2. Dane DS, Cameron CH, Briggs M. Virus-like particles in serum of patients with Australia-antigen-associated hepatitis. Lancet 1970;1:695–8.
3. Almeida JD, Rubenstein D, Stott EJ. New antigen-antibody system in Australia-antigen-positive hepatitis. Lancet 1971;2:1225–7.
4. Krugman S, Hoofnagle JH, Gerety RJ, et al. Viral hepatitis, type B, DNA polymerase activity and antibody to hepatitis B core antigen. N Engl J Med 1974; 290:1331–5.
5. Robinson WS. DNA and DNA polymerase in the core of the Dane particle of hepatitis B. Am J Med Sci 1975;270:151–9.
6. Galibert F, Mandart E, Fitoussi F, et al. Nucleotide sequence of the hepatitis B virus genome (subtype ayw) cloned in E. coli. Nature 1979;281:646–50.
7. Gibson UE, Heid CA, Williams PM. A novel method for real time quantitative RT-PCR. Genome Res 1996;6:995–1001.
8. Gordillo RM, Gutierrez J, Casal M. Evaluation of the COBAS TaqMan 48 real-time PCR system for quantitation of hepatitis B virus DNA. J Clin Microbiol 2005;43:3504–7.
9. Ranki M, Schatzl HM, Zachoval R, et al. Quantification of hepatitis B virus DNA over a wide range from serum for studying viral replicative activity in response to treatment and in recurrent infection. Hepatology 1995;21:1492–9.
10. Magnius LO, Espmark JA. New specificities in Australia antigen positive sera distinct from the Le Bouvier determinants. J Immunol 1972;109:1017–21.
11. Magnius LO. Characterization of a new antigen-antibody system associated with hepatitis B. Clin Exp Immuno 1975;20:209–16.

12. Alter HJ, Seeff LB, Kaplan PM, et al. Type B hepatitis: the infectivity of blood positive for e antigen and DNA polymerase after accidental needlestick exposure. N Engl J Med 1976;295:909–13.

13. Ohori H, Onodera S, Ishida N. Demonstration of hepatitis B e antigen (HBeAg) in association with intact Dane particles. J Gen Virol 1979;43:423–7.

14. Cappel R, DeCuyper F, Van F. Beers, e antigen and antibody, DNA polymerase, and inhibitors of DNA polymerase in acute and chronic hepatitis. J Infect Dis 1977;136:617–22.

15. Hindman SH, Gravelle CR, Murphy BL, et al. "e" Antigen, Dane particles, and serum DNA polymerase activity in HBsAg carriers. Ann Intern Med 1976;85:458–60.

16. Imai M, Tachibana FC, Moritsugu Y, et al. Hepatitis B antigen-associated deoxyribonucleic acid polymerase activity and e antigen/anti-e system. Infect Immun 1976;14:631–5.

17. Nordenfelt E, Kjellen L. Dane particles, DNA polymerase, and e-antigen in two different categories of hepatitis B antigen carriers. Intervirology 1975;5:225–32.

18. Takahashi K, Imai M, Tsuda F, et al. Association of dane particles with e antigen in the serum of asymptomatic carriers of hepatitis B surface antigen. J Immunol 1976;117:102–5.

19. Trepo C, Bird RG, Zuckerman AJ. Correlations between the detection of e antigen or antibody and electron microscopic pattern of hepatitis B surface antigen (HBsAg) associated particles in the serum of HBsAg carriers. J Clin Pathol 1977;30:216–20.

20. Werner BG, O'Connell AP, Summers J. Association of e antigen with Dane particle DNA in sera from asymptomatic carriers of hepatitis B surface antigen. Proc Natl Acad Sci U S A 1977;74:2149–51.

21. Trepo C, Vnek J, Prince AM. Delayed hypersensitivity and Arthus reaction to purified hepatitis B surface antigen (HBsAg) in immunized chimpanzees. Clin Immunol Immunopathol 1975;4:528–37.

22. Magnius LO, Lindholm A, Lundin P, et al. A new antigen-antibody system. Clinical significance in long-term carriers of hepatitis B surface antigen. JAMA 1975; 231:356–9.

23. Crosnier J, Jungers P, Courouce AM, et al. [Efficacy of a French hepatitis B vaccine. Results of a multicenter clinical trial, using a placebo, with double-blind randomized administration]. Bull Acad Natl Med 1980;164:764–76 [in French].

24. Maupas P, Chiron JP, Barin F, et al. Efficacy of hepatitis B vaccine in prevention of early HBsAg carrier state in children. Controlled trial in an endemic area (Senegal). Lancet 1981;1:289–92.

25. Szmuness W, Stevens CE, Harley EJ, et al. Hepatitis B vaccine: demonstration of efficacy in a controlled clinical trial in a high-risk population in the United States. N Engl J Med 1980;303:833–41.

26. Rendi-Wagner P, Kundi M, Stemberger H, et al. Antibody-response to three recombinant hepatitis B vaccines: comparative evaluation of multicenter travel-clinic based experience. Vaccine 2001;19:2055–60.

27. Zuckerman JN. Review: hepatitis B immune globulin for prevention of hepatitis B infection. J Med Virol 2007;79:919–21.

28. Chen DS, Hsu NH, Sung JL, et al. A mass vaccination program in Taiwan against hepatitis B virus infection in infants of hepatitis B surface antigen-carrier mothers. JAMA 1987;257:2597–603.

29. Beasley RP. Rocks along the road to the control of HBV and HCC. Ann Epidemiol 2009;19:231–4.

30. Liaw YF, Chu CM. Hepatitis B virus infection. Lancet 2009;373:582–92.

31. Chu CM, Karayiannis P, Fowler MJ, et al. Natural history of chronic hepatitis B virus infection in Taiwan: studies of hepatitis B virus DNA in serum. Hepatology 1985;5:431–4.
32. Chu CM, Liaw YF. Natural history differences in perinatally versus adult-acquired disease. Curr Hepat Rep 2004;3:123–31.
33. Liaw YF. Hepatitis flares and hepatitis B e antigen seroconversion: implication in anti-hepatitis B virus therapy. J Gastroenterol Hepatol 2003;18:246–52.
34. Chu CM, Hung SJ, Lin J, et al. Natural history of hepatitis B e antigen to antibody seroconversion in patients with normal serum aminotransferase levels. Am J Med 2004;116:829–34.
35. Hsu YS, Chien RN, Yeh CT, et al. Long-term outcome after spontaneous HBeAg seroconversion in patients with chronic hepatitis B. Hepatology 2002;35:1522–7.
36. Chen YC, Chu CM, Yeh CT, et al. Natural course following the onset of cirrhosis in patients with chronic hepatitis B: a long-term follow-up study. Hepatol Int 2007;1:267–73.
37. Chu CM, Liaw YF. HBsAg seroclearance in asymptomatic carriers of high endemic areas: appreciably high rates during a long-term follow-up. Hepatology 2007;45:1187–92.
38. Liaw YF, Sheen IS, Chen TJ, et al. Incidence, determinants and significance of delayed clearance of serum HBsAg in chronic hepatitis B virus infection: a prospective study. Hepatology 1991;13:627–31.
39. Yuen MF, Wong DK, Sablon E, et al. HBsAg seroclearance in chronic hepatitis B in the Chinese: virological, histological, and clinical aspects. Hepatology 2004; 39:1694–701.
40. Hadziyannis SJ, Lieberman HM, Karvountzis GG, et al. Analysis of liver disease, nuclear HBcAg, viral replication, and hepatitis B virus DNA in liver and serum of HBeAg Vs. anti-HBe positive carriers of hepatitis B virus. Hepatology 1983;3: 656–62.
41. Carman WF, Jacyna MR, Hadziyannis S, et al. Mutation preventing formation of hepatitis B e antigen in patients with chronic hepatitis B infection. Lancet 1989; 2:588–91.
42. Karayiannis P, Fowler MJ, Lok AS, et al. Detection of serum HBV-DNA by molecular hybridisation. Correlation with HBeAg/anti-HBe status, racial origin, liver histology and hepatocellular carcinoma. J Hepatol 1985;1:99–106.
43. Liaw YF, Tai DI, Chu CM, et al. The development of cirrhosis in patients with chronic type B hepatitis: a prospective study. Hepatology 1988;8:493–6.
44. Liaw YF, Tai DI, Chu CM, et al. Early detection of hepatocellular carcinoma in patients with chronic type B hepatitis. A prospective study. Gastroenterology 1986;90:263–7.
45. Chu CM, Liaw YF. Hepatitis B virus-related cirrhosis: natural history and treatment. Semin Liver Dis 2006;26:142–52.
46. Mason AL, Xu L, Guo L, et al. Molecular basis for persistent hepatitis B virus infection in the liver after clearance of serum hepatitis B surface antigen. Hepatology 1998;27:1736–42.
47. Chisari FV. Rous-Whipple Award Lecture. Viruses, immunity, and cancer: lessons from hepatitis B. Am J Pathol 2000;156:1117–32.
48. Wong DK, Cheung AM, O'Rourke K, et al. Effect of alpha-interferon treatment in patients with hepatitis B e antigen-positive chronic hepatitis B. A meta-analysis. Ann Intern Med 1993;119:312–23.
49. Lin SM, Sheen IS, Chien RN, et al. Long-term beneficial effect of interferon therapy in patients with chronic hepatitis B virus infection. Hepatology 1999;29:971–5.

50. Who U. WHO vaccine-preventable diseases: monitoring system. Global summary. WHO/IVB/2007 2007. Available at: http://whqlibdoc.who.int/hq/2007/WHO_IVB_2007_eng.pdf. Accesses December 15, 2010.
51. Ni YH, Huang LM, Chang MH, et al. Two decades of universal hepatitis B vaccination in Taiwan: impact and implication for future strategies. Gastroenterology 2007;132:1287–93.
52. Kao JH, Hsu HM, Shau WY, et al. Universal hepatitis B vaccination and the decreased mortality from fulminant hepatitis in infants in Taiwan. J Pediatr 2001;139:349–52.
53. Chen HL, Chang CJ, Kong MS, et al. Pediatric fulminant hepatic failure in endemic areas of hepatitis B infection: 15 years after universal hepatitis B vaccination. Hepatology 2004;39:58–63.
54. Namgyal P. Impact of hepatitis B immunization, Europe and worldwide. J Hepatol 2003;39(Suppl 1):77–82.
55. Chang MH, Chen CJ, Lai MS, et al. Universal hepatitis B vaccination in Taiwan and the incidence of hepatocellular carcinoma in children. Taiwan Childhood Hepatoma Study Group. N Engl J Med 1997;336:1855–9.
56. Chang MH, You SL, Chen CJ, et al. Decreased incidence of hepatocellular carcinoma in hepatitis B vaccinees: a 20-year follow-up study. J Natl Cancer Inst 2009;101:1348–55.
57. Chen CJ, Iloeje UH, Yang HI. Long-term outcomes in hepatitis B: the REVEAL-HBV study. Clin Liver Dis 2007;11:797–816, viii.
58. Chen CJ, Yang HI, Su J, et al. Risk of hepatocellular carcinoma across a biological gradient of serum hepatitis B virus DNA level. JAMA 2006;295:65–73.
59. Kao JH. Role of viral factors in the natural course and therapy of chronic hepatitis B. Hepatol Int 2007;1:415–30.
60. Chu CM, Liaw YF. Genotype C hepatitis B virus infection is associated with a higher risk of reactivation of hepatitis B and progression to cirrhosis than genotype B: a longitudinal study of hepatitis B e antigen-positive patients with normal aminotransferase levels at baseline. J Hepatol 2005;43:411–7.
61. Papatheodoridis GV, Chrysanthos N, Hadziyannis E, et al. Longitudinal changes in serum HBV DNA levels and predictors of progression during the natural course of HBeAg-negative chronic hepatitis B virus infection. J Viral Hepat 2008;15:434–41.
62. Hui CK, Leung N, Yuen ST, et al. Natural history and disease progression in Chinese chronic hepatitis B patients in immune-tolerant phase. Hepatology 2007;46:395–401.
63. Tai DI, Lin SM, Sheen IS, et al. Long-term outcome of hepatitis B e antigen-negative hepatitis B surface antigen carriers in relation to changes of alanine aminotransferase levels over time. Hepatology 2009;49:1859–67.
64. Chen YC, Sheen IS, Chu CM, et al. Prognosis following spontaneous HBsAg seroclearance in chronic hepatitis B patients with or without concurrent infection. Gastroenterology 2002;123:1084–9.
65. Tillmann HL, Hadem J, Leifeld L, et al. Safety and efficacy of lamivudine in patients with severe acute or fulminant hepatitis B, a multicenter experience. J Viral Hepat 2006;13:256–63.
66. Kim WR, Terrault NA, Pedersen RA, et al. Trends in waiting list registration for liver transplantation for viral hepatitis in the United States. Gastroenterology 2009;137:1680–6.
67. Lau GK. Hepatitis B reactivation after chemotherapy: two decades of clinical research. Hepatol Int 2008;2:152–62.

68. Samuel D, Muller R, Alexander G, et al. Liver transplantation in European patients with the hepatitis B surface antigen. N Engl J Med 1993;329:1842–7.
69. Fischer L, Sterneck M, Zollner B, et al. Lamivudine improves the prognosis of patients with hepatitis B after liver transplantation. Transplant Proc 2000;32:2128–30.
70. Gane EJ, Angus PW, Strasser S, et al. Lamivudine plus low-dose hepatitis B immunoglobulin to prevent recurrent hepatitis B following liver transplantation. Gastroenterology 2007;132:931–7.
71. Chien RN, Lin CH, Liaw YF. The effect of lamivudine therapy in hepatic decompensation during acute exacerbation of chronic hepatitis B. J Hepatol 2003;38:322–7.
72. Leung NW, Lai CL, Chang TT, et al. Extended lamivudine treatment in patients with chronic hepatitis B enhances hepatitis B e antigen seroconversion rates: results after 3 years of therapy. Hepatology 2001;33:1527–32.
73. Liaw YF, Chang TT, Wu SS, et al. Long-term entecavir therapy results in reversal of fibrosis/cirrhosis and continued histologic improvement in patients with HBeAg(+) and (-) chronic hepatitis B: results from studies ETV-022, -027 and -901. Hepatology 2008;48:706A.
74. Liaw YF, Sung JJ, Chow WC, et al. Lamivudine for patients with chronic hepatitis B and advanced liver disease. N Engl J Med 2004;351:1521–31.
75. Cooksley WG, Piratvisuth T, Lee SD, et al. Peginterferon alpha-2a (40 kDa): an advance in the treatment of hepatitis B e antigen-positive chronic hepatitis B. J Viral Hepat 2003;10:298–305.
76. Lau GK, Piratvisuth T, Luo KX, et al. Peginterferon Alfa-2a, lamivudine, and the combination for HBeAg-positive chronic hepatitis B. N Engl J Med 2005;352:2682–95.
77. Marcellin P, Lau GK, Bonino F, et al. Peginterferon alfa-2a alone, lamivudine alone, and the two in combination in patients with HBeAg-negative chronic hepatitis B. N Engl J Med 2004;351:1206–17.
78. Dan YY, Aung MO, Lim SG. The economics of treating chronic hepatitis B in Asia. Hepatol Int 2008;2:284–95.
79. Liaw YF. Antiviral therapy of chronic hepatitis B: opportunities and challenges in Asia. J Hepatol 2009;51:403–10.
80. Keeffe EB, Dieterich DT, Han SH, et al. A treatment algorithm for the management of chronic hepatitis B virus infection in the United States: 2008 update. Clin Gastroenterol Hepatol 2008;6:1315–41 [quiz: 1286].
81. European Association For The Study Of The Liver. EASL clinical practice guidelines: management of chronic hepatitis B. J Hepatol 2009;50:227–42.
82. Liaw YF, Leung N, Kao JH, et al. Asian-Pacific consensus statement on the management of chronic hepatitis B: a 2008 update. Hepatol Int 2008;2:263–83.
83. Lok AS, McMahon BJ. Chronic hepatitis B: update 2009. Hepatology 2009;50:661–2.
84. Kariv R, Leshno M, Beth-Or A, et al. Re-evaluation of serum alanine aminotransferase upper normal limit and its modulating factors in a large-scale population study. Liver Int 2006;26:445–50.
85. Prati D, Taioli E, Zanella A, et al. Updated definitions of healthy ranges for serum alanine aminotransferase levels. Ann Intern Med 2002;137:1–10.
86. Lai M, Hyatt BJ, Nasser I, et al. The clinical significance of persistently normal ALT in chronic hepatitis B infection. J Hepatol 2007;47:760–7.
87. Fung J, Lai CL, But D, et al. Prevalence of fibrosis and cirrhosis in chronic hepatitis B: implications for treatment and management. Hepatology 2007;46:647A.

88. Gui H, Xia Q, Wang H, et al. Predictors of significant histological findings in chronic hepatitis B patients with persistently normal ALT levels. Hepatology 2007;46:653A.

89. Nguyen MH, Trinh H, Garcia RT, et al. High prevalence of significant histologic disease in patients with chronic hepatitis B and normal ALT. Hepatology 2007; 46:680A.

90. Dumolard L, Gacic-Dobo M, Shapiro CN, et al; Centers for Disease Control and Prevention (CDC). Implementation of newborn hepatitis B vaccination—worldwide, 2006. MMWR Morb Mortal Wkly Rep 2008;57:1249–52.

91. Lin SY, Chang ET, So SK. Why we should routinely screen Asian American adults for hepatitis B: a cross-sectional study of Asians in California. Hepatology 2007; 46:1034–40.

92. Hann HW, Hann RS, Maddrey WC. Hepatitis B virus infection in 6,130 unvaccinated Korean-Americans surveyed between 1988 and 1990. Am J Gastroenterol 2007;102:767–72.

93. IOM. Hepatitis and liver cancer: a national strategy for prevention and control of hepatitis B and C. In: Colvin HM, Mitchell AE, editors. Washington, DC: The National Academies Press; 2009. p. 250.

94. Chien RN, Liaw YF. Nucleos(t)ide analogues for hepatitis B virus: strategies for long-term success. Best Pract Res Clin Gastroenterol 2008;22:1081–92.

95. Buti M, Brosa M, Casado MA, et al. Modeling the cost-effectiveness of different oral antiviral therapies in patients with chronic hepatitis B. J Hepatol 2009;51: 640–6.

96. Liaw YF. On-treatment outcome prediction and adjustment during chronic hepatitis B therapy: now and future. Antivir Ther 2009;14:13–22.

97. Keeffe EB, Zeuzem S, Koff RS, et al. Report of an international workshop: roadmap for management of patients receiving oral therapy for chronic hepatitis B. Clin Gastroenterol Hepatol 2007;5:890–7.

98. Werle-Lapostolle B, Bowden S, Locarnini S, et al. Persistence of cccDNA during the natural history of chronic hepatitis B and decline during adefovir dipivoxil therapy. Gastroenterology 2004;126:1750–8.

99. Peters M, Shouval D, Bonham A, et al. Posttransplantation: future therapies. Semin Liver Dis 2000;20(Suppl):S19–24.

100. Wands J, Geissler M, Putlitz J, et al. Nucleic acid-based antiviral and gene therapy of chronic hepatitis B infection. J Gastroenterol Hepatol 1997; 12(Suppl):S354–69.

Index

Note: Page numbers of article titles are in **boldface** type.

Clin Liver Dis 14 (2010) 547–553
doi:10.1016/S1089-3261(10)00055-3
1089-3261/10/$ – see front matter

Moving?

Make sure your subscription moves with you!

To notify us of your new address, find your **Clinics Account Number** (located on your mailing label above your name), and contact customer service at:

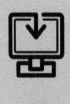

Email: journalscustomerservice-usa@elsevier.com

800-654-2452 (subscribers in the U.S. & Canada)
314-447-8871 (subscribers outside of the U.S. & Canada)

Fax number: 314-447-8029

Elsevier Health Sciences Division
Subscription Customer Service
3251 Riverport Lane
Maryland Heights, MO 63043

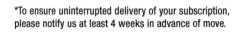

*To ensure uninterrupted delivery of your subscription, please notify us at least 4 weeks in advance of move.